3D Organoids and Stem Cells in Regenerative Endodontics

Mohammed Tarique and
Nezar Mohammed Boreak

CRC Press
Taylor & Francis Group
Boca Raton London New York

CRC Press is an imprint of the
Taylor & Francis Group, an **informa** business

Designed cover image: Shutterstock

First edition published 2027
by CRC Press
2385 NW Executive Center Drive, Suite 320, Boca Raton FL 33431

and by CRC Press
4 Park Square, Milton Park, Abingdon, Oxon, OX14 4RN

CRC Press is an imprint of Taylor & Francis Group, LLC

ISBN: 9781032964584 (hbk)
ISBN: 9781032964607 (pbk)
ISBN: 9781003589921 (ebk)

DOI: 10.1201/9781003589921

Typeset in Sabon
by codeMantra

Contents

Preface

Endodontic science has seen a decisive shift from biologically passive intervention to biologically active reconstruction of the dentin–pulp complex. This transition has been driven by advances in stem cell biology, ECM engineering, microenvironmental modulation, and high-fidelity 3D culture systems. This book reviews the latest developments in regenerative endodontics, linking molecular regulation, engineered scaffolds, cell–matrix interactions, and advanced biofabrication technologies to the mechanistic processes underlying dental tissue regeneration.

Chapter 1 establishes the biological and translational context for regenerative endodontics by delineating the molecular composition, immunological functions, and structural constraints of the native dentin–pulp complex. It presents the current understanding of stem-cell recruitment, niche signaling, and the limitations inherent to conventional devitalizing procedures.

Chapters 2 and 3 extend this framework into 3D culture systems in dental regeneration. Organoid technologies presented in Chapter 2 demonstrate the role of multicellular, self-organized structures that recapitulate odontoblast–fibroblast–endothelial interactions, inflammatory signaling dynamics, and matrix deposition patterns that cannot be modeled in planar systems. Chapter 3 examines bioprinting modalities with an emphasis on bioink rheology, spatial fidelity, multimaterial printing, and their relevance for constructing anatomically constrained pulp geometries. Collectively, these chapters outline the 3D systems that provide both mechanistic insight and translational feasibility.

Chapter 4 focuses on scaffolds as structural and biochemical regulators of cell behavior. It examines natural and synthetic matrices in terms of porosity, degradation kinetics, ligand presentation, viscoelasticity, and their influence on odontogenic lineage commitment. Scaffold microarchitecture is linked explicitly to cell polarization, angiogenic patterning, and the directional deposition of dentin-like matrices, providing a materials-science perspective essential for rational design.

Chapters 5 and 6 address the biological effectors that govern tissue formation. Chapter 5 characterizes dental stem cell populations, exploring their transcriptomic signatures, differentiation trajectories, and responsiveness to mechanical and biochemical stimuli. Chapter 6 builds upon this with an analysis of extracellular vesicles as nanoscale carriers of mRNA, microRNA, and protein cargo that modulate odontogenesis, neurotrophic signaling, angiogenesis, and immune resolution.

Chapter 7 integrates the immunological dimension, emphasizing the temporal and phenotypic transitions of macrophages, neutrophil dynamics, cytokine gradients, and the molecular determinants that distinguish reparative from destructive inflammation. It highlights the immune–stem-cell crosstalk that governs scaffold integration, vascular ingrowth, and the quality of neo-tissue formed within the canal space.

The volume culminates in Chapter 8, which synthesizes the molecular signals that coordinate these diverse biological processes. Signaling axes, including Wnt/β-catenin, BMP–Smad, TGF-β–Smad, PI3K–AKT–mTOR, and Notch, are examined as interconnected regulatory systems that drive transcriptional activation, lineage specification, angiogenic induction, and matrix organization. These pathways provide the mechanistic backbone that unifies the cellular, biomaterial, and immunological themes presented throughout the preceding chapters.

This book presents regenerative endodontics as a coherent, mechanistically defined field rooted in reproducible biological principles and supported by convergent evidence across molecular, cellular, materials, and engineering sciences. The compilation is intended as a reference for researchers and graduate-level scholars seeking a conceptually integrated understanding of the processes that govern the reconstruction of the dentin–pulp complex.

About the Authors

Mohammed Tarique is a researcher and academic with expertise in molecular biology, biotechnology, and nanomedicine, working at Jamia Islamia. He is a founder and Director of Almanac Life Science India Private Limited, India. He earned his PhD from the International Centre for Genetic Engineering and Biotechnology (ICGEB), New Delhi, and has conducted postdoctoral research in parasite cell biology. He is a member of several editorial boards. His research is published in high-impact journals, and he holds patents related to diabetic neuropathy treatment and glucose monitoring devices. Additionally, he has authored books on nanomedicine applications in cancer diagnosis and therapy, as well as the use of nanoparticles in tissue engineering and infectious diseases.

Nezar Mohammed Boreak is an academic and researcher specializing in the applications of stem cells and 3D organoids in endodontics. He earned his PhD in Dental Sciences and Clinical Certificate in Endodontics from Tohoku University, Japan, and furthered his expertise with a Certificate in Dental Implantology and the American Board in Implantology from New York University (NYU), USA. Currently, he serves as an Associate Professor and Consultant in Restorative Dentistry (Endodontics), College of Dentistry, Jazan University, Saudi Arabia. He earned his Doctor of Philosophy (PhD) in Endodontics from Tohoku University, Japan, and is American Board-certified in Implant Dentistry from New York University, USA.

He previously served as Head of the Department, Vice Dean for Academic Affairs, and Head of the Alumni Unit. He is currently a member of the Curriculum Development Committee. He also served as the regional representative of the Saudi Endodontic Society in the Jazan Region and as the ICOI representative in Saudi Arabia. He is actively involved in teaching, clinical practice, research, and academic leadership in Endodontics and Restorative Dentistry.

Chapter 1

Introduction to regenerative endodontics

1.1 INTRODUCTION

Regenerative endodontics is an emerging field in dental science that integrates principles of tissue engineering to restore the biological function and structure of the pulp–dentin complex. Unlike conventional endodontic therapy, which primarily focuses on disinfection and mechanical debridement followed by obturation with inert materials, regenerative endodontic procedures (REPs) aim to revive biological activity within the root canal system by leveraging the body's innate regenerative potential. The American Association of Endodontists (AAE) defines regenerative endodontics as biologically based procedures designed to replace damaged structures, including dentin and root structures, as well as cells of the pulp–dentin complex (AAE, 2021). This definition underscores a fundamental shift in the approach to endodontic treatment, moving from symptom-based intervention toward true tissue regeneration.

The foundation of regenerative endodontics lies in the principles of tissue engineering, which involve a triad of components, namely, stem cells, scaffolds, and bioactive molecules. These elements work in unison to promote the repopulation of the root canal system with vital cells, ultimately leading to the formation of new pulp-like tissue capable of responding to physiological stimuli. Stem cells, particularly those derived from the apical papilla (SCAP), dental pulp (DPSCs), and periodontal ligament (PDLSCs), play a critical role in this process. SCAP, which reside at the apices of immature teeth, are particularly crucial in the regenerative process due to their high proliferative potential and ability to differentiate into odontoblast-like cells responsible for dentinogenesis (Kim et al., 2018). These stem cells interact with bioactive molecules such as bone morphogenetic proteins (BMPs), vascular endothelial growth factors (VEGF), and platelet-derived growth factors (PDGF), which orchestrate cellular differentiation and angiogenesis, ensuring the formation of a functional vascular network within the newly regenerated pulp (Galler et al., 2020).

The scope of regenerative endodontics has significantly expanded over the past decade, evolving from its initial application in immature permanent teeth

DOI: 10.1201/9781003589921-1

with necrotic pulp to broader indications that include pulp revitalization in mature teeth and experimental approaches in whole-tooth regeneration. Immature permanent teeth with necrotic pulp historically presented a significant clinical challenge since conventional treatment options, such as calcium hydroxide apexification or mineral trioxide aggregate (MTA) apical barriers, failed to support continued root development, leaving teeth vulnerable to fracture (Torabinejad and Nosrat, 2019). REPs have since emerged as a superior alternative by facilitating continued root maturation through endogenous tissue regeneration. Clinical studies have consistently demonstrated that REPs promote increased root length and dentinal wall thickness, reducing the likelihood of root fractures and restoring some degree of pulp vitality (Murray, 2023). This outcome is achieved by inducing a controlled inflammatory response, which triggers the recruitment of endogenous stem cells from periapical tissues into the disinfected canal space, where they differentiate into odontoblast-like cells capable of depositing new dentin.

In addition to its application in immature teeth, regenerative endodontics has been investigated for its potential use in mature teeth with necrotic pulp. Although mature teeth lack an open apical foramen that facilitates stem cell recruitment, studies have explored alternative approaches such as exogenous stem cell transplantation, growth factor delivery, and scaffold-based tissue engineering. Experimental evidence suggests that the controlled introduction of DPSCs into a suitable biomimetic scaffold, combined with signaling molecules like transforming growth factor-beta (TGF-β), can promote partial regeneration of pulp-like tissue in mature teeth (Zhou et al., 2023). While the clinical feasibility of such procedures remains under investigation, these findings indicate the possibility of extending regenerative techniques beyond their traditional indications.

A key component of regenerative endodontics is the development of biocompatible scaffolds that support cellular migration, adhesion, and differentiation within the root canal space. Traditionally, blood clot formation has been used as a natural scaffold in regenerative procedures, relying on induced bleeding from periapical tissues to create a fibrin-rich matrix conducive to cellular proliferation. However, newer biomaterial-based scaffolds have demonstrated superior outcomes by offering enhanced control over the spatial organization and differentiation of regenerating tissues. Hydrogel-based scaffolds enriched with growth factors, electrospun nanofiber matrices, and 3D-printed bioactive scaffolds have all been explored as potential alternatives to blood clot scaffolds, improving both the predictability and success of regenerative procedures (Liu et al., 2022). These materials not only provide structural support but also enable controlled release of bioactive molecules, ensuring sustained stimulation of stem cell differentiation throughout the regenerative process.

Despite the promising advancements in regenerative endodontics, several challenges remain. One of the primary limitations is the inconsistency in clinical outcomes, which can be attributed to variations in patient biology, infection control, and procedural protocols. Unlike traditional endodontic therapy, which follows well-established protocols, regenerative procedures involve a dynamic biological response that can be influenced by factors such as the severity of infection, the presence of residual bacteria, and the patient's immune response (Murray et al., 2021). Additionally, the long-term viability of regenerated pulp-like tissue remains a topic of ongoing investigation. While histological studies have confirmed the presence of newly formed connective tissue and vascular structures within the root canal, the extent to which this tissue retains full functional properties comparable to those of native pulp is still uncertain (Diogenes et al., 2023).

Future research in regenerative endodontics is likely to focus on refining biomaterial technologies, optimizing stem cell delivery mechanisms, and exploring gene-editing techniques to enhance the efficiency and reliability of tissue regeneration. Gene therapy, particularly CRISPR-based approaches, has been proposed to modify stem cell behavior, enhance regenerative potential, and improve the immune compatibility of implanted cells. Additionally, advances in 3D bioprinting have raised the possibility of creating patient-specific pulp tissue constructs that can be implanted into root canals, further expanding the clinical applicability of regenerative endodontic therapies (Shah and Loghin, 2021).

1.2 SIGNIFICANCE OF REGENERATIVE ENDODONTICS

Traditional endodontic treatments, particularly root canal therapy (RCT), have long been the gold standard for managing irreversible pulpitis and necrotic pulp. These procedures involve mechanical debridement, chemical disinfection, and subsequent obturation of the root canal space with inert materials to prevent reinfection. While RCT has proven to be highly successful in eliminating infection and preserving the structural integrity of the tooth, it comes with inherent biological limitations (Table 1.1). The removal of the pulp tissue, which houses vascular, immune, and neurosensory components, leaves the tooth in a devitalized state, depriving it of the ability to respond to physiological stimuli, repair itself, or mount an effective defense against future injury (Torabinejad and Nosrat, 2019). The resulting tooth, though structurally intact, becomes more brittle over time due to the loss of internal hydration and proprioceptive feedback mechanisms, increasing susceptibility to fracture and functional deterioration (Murray et al., 2021).

Regenerative endodontics presents an advanced therapeutic paradigm that moves beyond conventional infection control to emphasize the biologically driven reconstruction and functional restoration of the dentin–pulp complex. Unlike conventional RCT, regenerative procedures aim to repopulate the root canal space with functional pulp-like tissue that restores vascularity, innervation, and immunocompetence. This advancement has profound

Table 1.1 Comparison of regenerative endodontics and traditional root canal therapy (RCT)

Feature	*Regenerative endodontics (REPs)*	*Traditional root canal therapy*
Objective	Tissue regeneration and pulp revitalization	Disinfection and obturation
Pulp status	Restores pulp-like tissue	Nonvital, devitalized tooth
Root development	Allows continued root growth	No further root maturation
Mechanical preparation	Minimal or no instrumentation	Extensive canal shaping
Disinfection method	Low-concentration irrigants and bioactive medicaments	High-concentration NaOCl and mechanical debridement
Long-term strength	Increased dentin thickness and resilience	Increased fracture susceptibility
Clinical success rate	Promising but variable	Well-established and predictable

implications for long-term dental health as the revitalized pulp can maintain homeostasis, repair minor injuries, and support continued root development in cases of immature teeth with open apices (Kim et al., 2018). The capacity to regenerate pulp tissue enables a fundamental shift in clinical management, whereby pulp necrosis is no longer regarded as an irreversibly degenerative state requiring permanent devitalization. Instead, clinicians can pursue biologically based interventions aimed at re-establishing a viable, vascularized, and sensory-responsive tissue system within the root canal.

One of the major advantages of regenerative endodontics is its capacity to improve the structural integrity of treated teeth. Regenerative procedures have demonstrated the ability to promote continued dentin deposition, leading to increased root wall thickness and, consequently, enhanced overall biomechanical stability. (Murray, 2023). Histological studies have confirmed that, following regenerative procedures, newly formed dentin and pulp-like connective tissue contribute to structural reinforcement, mitigating the risk of catastrophic failures commonly associated with conventionally treated nonvital teeth (Zhou et al., 2023). This is particularly relevant in young patients with necrotic immature teeth, where continued root development is crucial for long-term tooth retention. Traditional apexification procedures, which induce the formation of a calcified barrier at the root apex, do not contribute to root elongation or thickening of dentinal walls. In contrast, regenerative procedures leverage endogenous stem cell activity to promote natural root maturation, ultimately yielding a more resilient tooth structure (Galler et al., 2020).

Beyond structural benefits, regenerative endodontics also restores the biological function of the pulp, reintroducing vascularization and innervation within the root canal system. The presence of newly formed blood vessels ensures the delivery of nutrients and immune cells, enhancing the tooth's ability to respond to bacterial challenges, repair micro-damage, and maintain overall homeostasis (Diogenes et al., 2023). Revascularized pulp tissue can potentially modulate the inflammatory response, reducing the likelihood of secondary infections and post-treatment complications. Additionally, the restoration of proprioceptive nerve fibers within the pulp–dentin complex allows the tooth to regain its ability to detect occlusal forces and external stimuli, thereby improving functional integration within the dentition (Zhang et al., 2023).

Another critical aspect of the significance of regenerative endodontics lies in its potential to extend the lifespan of teeth. Traditional RCT, although effective, has been associated with a gradual decline in long-term survival rates, particularly in cases where substantial structural damage is observed at the time of treatment. Studies have shown that endodontically treated teeth, especially in high-load-bearing areas, are more likely to undergo restorative failures or require extraction due to secondary fractures (Murray et al., 2021). Regenerative procedures, by contrast, may offer a means of improving tooth longevity by preserving its biological function and promoting tissue repair. The preservation of a viable, responsive pulp promotes superior integration with restorative materials, lowers the likelihood of coronal microleakage, and sustains physiological aging processes that collectively support long-term dental health.

Regenerative endodontics is also significant from clinical and patient-centered viewpoints. Although conventional RCT achieves high success rates, it is often burdened by negative patient perceptions, largely due to postoperative discomfort and the idea of retaining a nonvital (Shah and Loghin, 2021). The prospect of revitalizing a tooth rather than simply disinfecting and sealing it aligns with patient expectations for more natural and biologically sustainable treatments. Furthermore, advancements in regenerative techniques have the potential to simplify procedures by reducing the reliance on complex retreatment strategies in cases of endodontic failure. Instead of retreating failed root canals, clinicians may ultimately be able to employ regenerative approaches to re-establish functional pulp tissue, thereby reducing the need for tooth extraction or subsequent prosthetic rehabilitation (Galler et al., 2020).

1.3 BIOLOGICAL BASIS OF REGENERATIVE ENDODONTICS

Regenerative endodontics is fundamentally rooted in the principles of tissue engineering, which harnesses the biological mechanisms of cell proliferation, differentiation, and extracellular matrix (ECM) organization to restore the dentin–pulp complex. It aims to reconstitute the pulp tissue, re-establish vascularization, and support dentinogenesis. The success of pulp regeneration depends on three essential components: stem/progenitor cells, growth factors, and scaffolds, which collectively create a conducive microenvironment for tissue repair and functional restoration (Diogenes and Ruparel, 2017). These elements interact in a dynamic process, mimicking natural wound healing and developmental biology to facilitate regeneration within the root canal system (Figure 1.1).

The role of stem cells in regenerative endodontics is central to the process of pulp–dentin regeneration. Stem cells possess self-renewal capabilities and the potential to differentiate into multiple cell lineages, including odontoblast-like cells responsible for dentin formation. Several dental-derived mesenchymal stem cell populations have been identified as key players in pulp regeneration. Among these, DPSCs constitute a well-characterized population distinguished by strong proliferative capacity and broad multipotent differentiation potential (Galler et al., 2020). These cells reside within the perivascular niche of the pulp and are capable of differentiating into odontoblast-like cells under appropriate stimuli, contributing to dentin matrix deposition. Another critical stem cell population is stem cells derived from the apical papilla, which are particularly important in immature permanent teeth. SCAP demonstrate a high proliferative

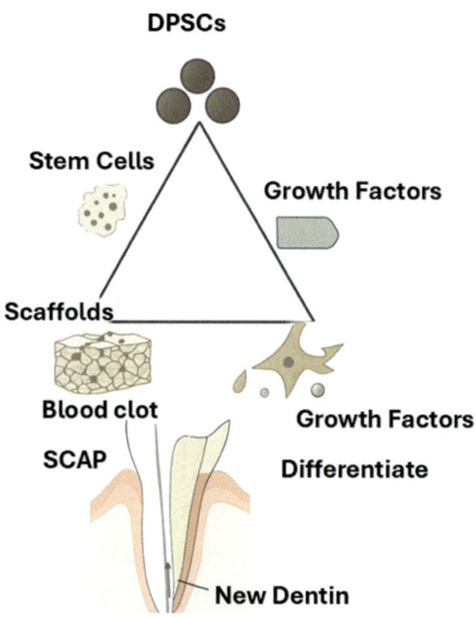

Figure 1.1 Tissue engineering triad in regenerative endodontics. Stem cells, scaffolds, and growth factors. Stem/progenitor cells such as DPSCs, SCAP, and PDLSCs interact with scaffolds including blood clots, collagen matrices, or hydrogels. Growth factors such as TGF-β, VEGF, and BMPs regulate cell homing, angiogenesis, and odontoblastic differentiation.

capacity and the ability to undergo odontogenic differentiation, making them important for continued root development and repair in regenerative procedures (Figure 1.2) (Kim et al., 2018). Additionally, PDLSCs and bone marrow-derived mesenchymal stem cells have been explored as alternative sources for pulp regeneration, although their functional integration within the dentin–pulp complex remains an area of ongoing research (Bakhtiar et al., 2017). The recruitment of endogenous stem cells from periapical tissues following the induction of controlled inflammation plays a fundamental role in the success of regenerative treatments as these cells migrate into the root canal and repopulate the scaffold environment.

In addition to stem cells, growth factors and signaling molecules function as essential regulators that coordinate the proliferation, migration, and differentiation of cells involved in the regenerative process. Growth factors are bioactive molecules that regulate cell behavior by binding to specific receptors and triggering intracellular signaling cascades. TGF-β plays a pivotal role in pulp regeneration by modulating odontoblast differentiation and ECM production (Murray, 2023). TGF-β also contributes to the immune modulation required for successful regenerative outcomes, influencing macrophage polarization and mitigating excessive inflammatory responses that could compromise tissue integration. The essential signaling molecules, bone morphogenetic proteins, particularly BMP-2 and

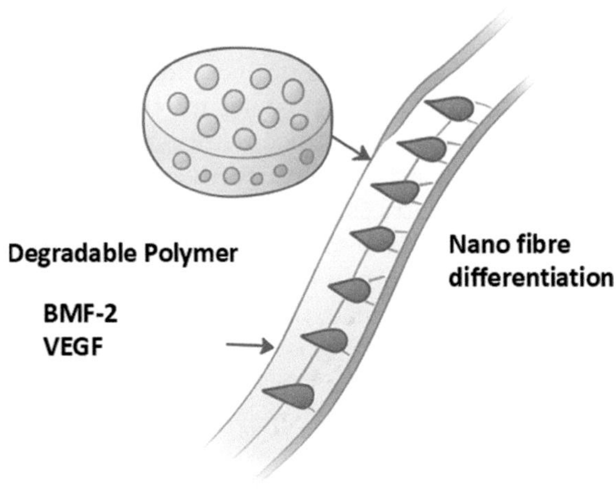

Figure 1.2 Functional role of stem cells from the apical papilla in regenerative endodontics. SCAP migrate into the disinfected canal following induction of bleeding, differentiate into odontoblast-like cells under the influence of BMPs and TGF-β, and deposit new dentin that contributes to continued root elongation and thickening of dentinal walls.

BMP-7, have been shown to promote odontoblastic differentiation and dentinogenesis (Zhou et al., 2023). These factors interact with cellular receptors to activate Smad-dependent pathways, enhancing the production of collagenous and noncollagenous proteins involved in the formation of reparative dentin. VEGF is a critical mediator in pulp regeneration as it promotes angiogenesis within the developing tissue, thereby establishing the blood supply required for cell survival, oxygen delivery, and nutrient transport (Zhang et al., 2023). Inadequate vascularization leaves newly formed tissues vulnerable to ischemia and necrosis, emphasizing the importance of optimizing VEGF-mediated angiogenic activity in regenerative endodontic strategies.

The third critical component in regenerative endodontics is the scaffold, which provides a three-dimensional matrix that supports cell attachment, migration, and organization within the root canal space (Figure 1.1). Scaffolds act as an ECM, allowing for the retention of regenerative cells and bioactive molecules in the canal environment. The most traditional scaffold used in regenerative endodontics is the blood clot, induced through the creation of periapical bleeding during revascularization procedures (Murray et al., 2021). The fibrin network formed within the blood clot serves as a natural scaffold that supports cell adhesion and growth factor retention. However, due to the variability and unpredictability associated with blood clot formation, alternative scaffold materials have been explored. Collagen-based scaffolds derived from natural ECM components offer biocompatibility and promote cellular migration and differentiation. These scaffolds mimic the native pulp ECM, providing an environment conducive to tissue regeneration. In addition, hydrogel-based scaffolds, composed of biomaterials such as hyaluronic acid and chitosan, have demonstrated enhanced bioactivity by allowing for the controlled release of growth factors and cellular guidance cues (Abbass et al., 2020). Advances in electrospun nanofiber scaffolds have further improved the structural properties of regenerative matrices, creating a biomimetic architecture that closely resembles the natural pulp–dentin interface. More recently, 3D bioprinting has been applied to scaffold fabrication, enabling the generation of patient-specific, pulp-like constructs that incorporate viable cells and spatially regulated, controlled-release bioactive molecules, thereby advancing the precision and biological fidelity of regenerative endodontic applications (Diogenes et al., 2023).

The interplay between stem cells, growth factors, and scaffolds determines the success of REPs (Figure 1.1). The recruitment of endogenous or transplanted stem cells into a bioactive microenvironment enriched with growth factors ensures their differentiation into odontoblast-like cells capable of dentin secretion. The scaffold, in turn, provides the necessary mechanical and biological cues that guide tissue organization, ensuring functional integration of regenerated pulp. However, several challenges remain in optimizing this regenerative triad to achieve consistent clinical outcomes. The variability in patient-specific stem cell responses, the risk of bacterial contamination, and the unpredictability of tissue differentiation highlight the need for continued refinement of regenerative protocols (Torabinejad and Nosrat, 2019). Future research is likely to focus on the development of smart biomaterials capable of dynamically responding to cellular needs, as well as the incorporation of gene-editing technologies to enhance stem cell function and immune compatibility.

1.4 CURRENT CLINICAL PROTOCOLS IN REGENERATIVE ENDODONTICS

Regenerative endodontics has gained widespread clinical acceptance as a biologically driven approach for managing necrotic immature permanent teeth, offering an alternative to traditional apexification or RCT. The contemporary protocols employed in REPs are designed to create an optimal environment for endogenous stem cell recruitment, proliferation, and differentiation, ultimately leading to the regeneration of pulp-like tissue within the root canal. The main steps in the standard procedure comprise minimal mechanical instrumentation, effective chemical disinfection, intracanal medication, controlled induction of bleeding, and biocompatible sealing to support tissue formation. While these steps have been refined over the past decade, variations exist in clinical execution based on factors such as patient age, extent of root development, and clinician preference (Diogenes and Ruparel, 2017). Each of these steps is described below and presented in Figure 1.3.

The first step in a regenerative protocol is disinfection of the root canal system, a critical process that must balance antimicrobial efficacy with the preservation of residual viable stem cells within the dentin and periapical tissues (Table 1.2). Unlike conventional RCT, where mechanical debridement is a primary method for eliminating microbial biofilms, REPs rely heavily on chemical disinfection to avoid excessive damage to remaining stem cell niches. Sodium hypochlorite (NaOCl) is the most commonly used irritant, though its concentration is significantly reduced (typically 1.5%–3%) compared to traditional endodontic therapy, where higher concentrations (5.25%) are used (Torabinejad and Nosrat, 2019). The rationale for using lower concentrations is to minimize cytotoxicity to apical stem cells while still achieving sufficient bacterial decontamination. Studies have shown that higher concentrations of NaOCl can adversely affect stem cell viability, reducing their ability to adhere to dentin and differentiate into odontoblast-like cells (Galler et al., 2020). In many protocols, irrigation is supplemented with ethylenediaminetetraacetic acid (EDTA), typically at 17% concentration, which plays a crucial role in modulating dentin surface

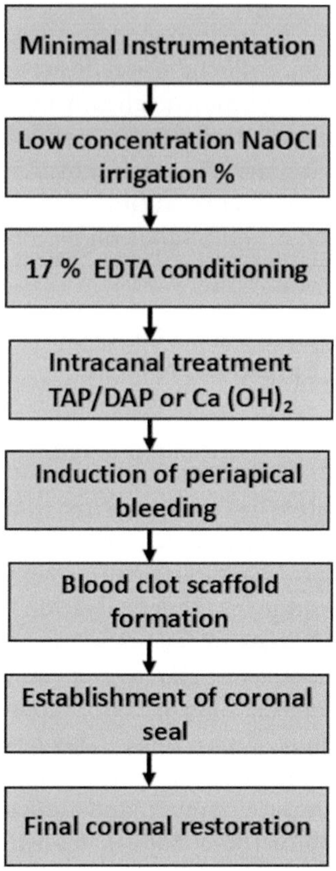

Figure 1.3 Stepwise clinical protocol for REPs. Following conservative preparation, the canal is disinfected using low-strength NaOCl and EDTA, medicated, and subsequently filled with a blood clot scaffold induced by apical irritation. A bioceramic material seals the clot coronally, enabling stem cell homing and continued root development.

properties to enhance stem cell attachment. EDTA removes the smear layer, exposes dentinal tubules, and releases embedded bioactive molecules such as TGF-β, which are instrumental in signaling stem cell differentiation and dentin matrix formation (Zhang et al., 2023).

Following disinfection, an intracanal bioactive agent is placed to suppress residual microbial activity and enhance the regenerative potential of the canal space. Two commonly used medicaments are triple antibiotic paste (TAP) and calcium hydroxide ($Ca(OH)_2$). TAP, which consists of ciprofloxacin, metronidazole, and minocycline, has been widely used due to its broad-spectrum antimicrobial action against anaerobic and facultative bacteria commonly found in necrotic pulp tissues (Murray, 2023). However, concerns regarding the potential cytotoxic effects of TAP on stem cells have

Table 1.2 Regenerative endodontic procedure overview

Step	*Procedure*	*Purpose*	*Common materials used*
Disinfection	Minimal instrumentation and gentle irrigation	Remove bacteria while preserving stem cells	1.5% NaOCl, 17% EDTA, and chlorhexidine (CHX)
Intracanal medicament	Placement of antibacterial medicament	Eliminate residual bacteria	TAP, DAP, and $Ca(OH)_2$
Induction of bleeding	Mechanical irritation of periapical tissues	Provide a natural scaffold with growth factors	Apical over-instrumentation
Sealing the canal	Placement of a biocompatible coronal barrier	Prevent contamination and support regeneration	MTA, biodentine, and bioceramics
Final restoration	Permanent coronal seal	Prevent bacterial re-entry	Composite resin and glass ionomer

led to modifications in its concentration and alternative formulations, such as double antibiotic paste (DAP), which excludes minocycline to prevent dentin discoloration. Alternatively, $Ca(OH)_2$ is favored for its ability to create an alkaline environment that promotes hard tissue deposition while also exerting antimicrobial effects. While both intracanal materials are clinically effective, evidence indicates that $Ca(OH)_2$ exerts a comparatively lower inhibitory effect on stem cell viability than TAP, making it the preferable choice when aiming to optimize regenerative potential (Zhou et al., 2023).

Once the intracanal material has remained in place for 1–4 weeks, depending on the severity of infection, it is removed with copious irrigation, after which the next phase is initiated, namely, the induction of bleeding into the canal space. This step is essential for generating a natural scaffold enriched with stem cells originating from the apical papilla, periapical tissues, and circulating progenitor cells. Bleeding is induced by extending a sterile endodontic file or instrument beyond the apical foramen, thereby stimulating the periapical tissues and allowing blood to enter and fill the canal space (Kim et al., 2018). The formation of a blood clot within the root canal provides a fibrin-rich matrix that acts as a natural scaffold for stem cell adhesion, migration, and proliferation. The blood clot also contains PDGF, VEGF, and TGF-β, which are critical for stimulating angiogenesis and cell differentiation (Bakhtiar et al., 2017). The clot is typically formed 1–3 mm below the cementoenamel junction (CEJ) to allow space for the subsequent placement of a biocompatible sealing material.

Following stabilization of the blood clot, a coronal seal is established using a bioactive material such as mineral trioxide aggregate (MTA) or newer bioceramic formulations. MTA remains the gold standard, supported by extensive evidence demonstrating its excellent biocompatibility, superior sealing capacity, and its ability to induce hard tissue formation (Torabinejad and Nosrat, 2019). In regenerative endodontics, its primary role is to function as a mechanical and biological barrier between the clot and definitive restoration, preventing bacterial ingress while simultaneously promoting mineralized tissue deposition (Figure 1.3). Bioceramic alternatives such as biodentine and EndoSequence Root Repair Material (ERRM) have also gained prominence, offering favorable handling characteristics and accelerated setting times compared with traditional MTA. These materials release calcium ions that enhance osteogenic and dentinogenic differentiation, thereby further supporting the formation of pulp-like tissue. Once the coronal barrier is established, a definitive composite or glass ionomer restoration is placed to achieve a hermetic seal, thereby preventing bacterial penetration and safeguarding the long-term success of the regenerative procedure. (Murray et al., 2021).

The overarching aim of regenerative protocols is to establish conditions that support stem cell homing and differentiation, enabling the formation of vascularized, pulp-like tissue that can sustain continued root development. Histological evaluations of successful cases reveal that the tissues formed within the canal vary considerably, ranging from vascularized connective tissue to odontoblast-like cells capable of generating new dentin (Diogenes et al., 2023). Nonetheless, outcome variability remains a major clinical challenge, with some cases showing limited regeneration or incomplete root maturation. Regenerative predictability is influenced by several factors, including patient age, stage of root development, extent of periapical pathology, and procedural variables. Younger patients with open apices and a more abundant SCAP population typically demonstrate more consistent and favorable outcomes than older individuals with reduced regenerative capacity (Galler et al., 2020).

While regenerative endodontics continue to advance, several refinements to existing protocols are under investigation to improve treatment predictability. Emerging bioactive scaffolds, such as synthetic hydrogels, collagen-based matrices, and electrospun nanofibers, present promising alternatives to conventional blood clot scaffolds by offering more controlled architectures that support consistent cell adhesion, migration, and tissue integration. In parallel, systems for controlled growth factor delivery and experimental gene-editing strategies, including CRISPR-mediated enhancement of stem cell function, are being explored as potential approaches to further optimize regenerative outcomes in the coming years (Shah and Loghin, 2021).

The standardization of regenerative endodontic protocols marks an important advancement toward integrating biologically based therapies into routine clinical practice. Through the optimization of disinfection methods, the development of more sophisticated scaffold systems, and the refinement of bioactive material applications, regenerative endodontics is positioned to transform the management of necrotic teeth by providing a biologically sustainable, long-term alternative to conventional endodontic treatment.

1.5 CLINICAL OUTCOMES AND CHALLENGES IN REGENERATIVE ENDODONTICS

REPs have shown encouraging clinical results, providing a biologically based alternative to conventional RCT by facilitating true regeneration of the dentin–pulp complex. In contrast to traditional approaches that yield a permanently devitalized tooth, regenerative techniques aim to re-establish vascularity, neurosensory capacity, and ongoing root maturation. Accumulating clinical evidence supports several favorable outcomes, including resolution of periapical radiolucencies, continued root development, increased dentinal wall thickness, and the formation of pulp-like tissue within the canal space (Diogenes et al., 2023).

Despite these advantages, important limitations persist, such as variability in patient response, esthetic challenges including treatment-related discoloration, and the absence of universally accepted clinical protocols. Addressing these issues is essential to improving predictability and facilitating broader integration of regenerative endodontics into routine clinical practice.

Clinical studies have consistently reported that REPs lead to significant periapical healing, with the resolution of radiolucencies occurring in a high percentage of treated cases (Torabinejad and Nosrat, 2019). This suggests that regenerative therapies not only promote pulp tissue formation but also effectively manage periapical infections. The increase in root length and thickening of dentinal walls observed in successfully treated cases is a major advantage over apexification techniques, which only induce the formation of a mineralized apical barrier without allowing further root elongation (Galler et al., 2020). Several longitudinal studies have confirmed that regenerative procedures in immature teeth lead to measurable gains in both root length and thickness over time, thereby enhancing the biomechanical stability of the treated tooth and reducing fracture susceptibility (Murray, 2023).

However, one of the primary challenges in regenerative endodontics is the variability in clinical outcomes. The success of REPs depends on multiple factors, including the patient's age, the type of tooth being treated, the degree of infection, and the specific protocol used. Younger patients with immature teeth tend to exhibit better outcomes as their apical papilla contains a higher population of stem cells that can be recruited for regeneration (Kim et al., 2018). Conversely, older patients or those with closed apices often show less predictable results due to the limited availability of endogenous stem cells in the periapical region (Zhou et al., 2023). Additionally, the extent of periapical infection plays a critical role in determining the success of regenerative procedures. Severe infections with large periapical lesions may compromise the ability of stem cells to survive and integrate within the canal space, reducing the likelihood of achieving complete regeneration (Zhang et al., 2023).

Another important limitation of regenerative endodontics is tooth discoloration, which is most commonly linked to the use of specific intracanal materials and certain coronal sealing agents. TAP, which contains minocycline, is known to cause intrinsic staining of dentin, particularly in anterior teeth where esthetic concerns are paramount (Diogenes and Ruparel, 2017). To mitigate this issue, alternative formulations such as DAP, which excludes minocycline, or $Ca(OH)_2$-based medicaments have been investigated as viable substitutes (Murray et al., 2021). Additionally, MTA, a commonly used sealing material in REPs, has been associated with tooth discoloration due to its bismuth oxide content. To address this concern, newer bioceramic materials such as Biodentine and ERRM have been introduced as alternatives that offer comparable bioactivity without the risk of significant discoloration (Shah and Loghin, 2021).

A major limitation in regenerative endodontics is the absence of fully standardized clinical protocols. Although broad treatment recommendations are available, substantial variability persists in the selection of irrigants, intracanal materials, scaffold systems, and coronal sealing techniques across studies and clinical environments (Torabinejad and Nosrat, 2019). This heterogeneity complicates the comparison of treatment outcomes and hinders the development of universally accepted best practices. For example, although lower concentrations of NaOCl are favored to reduce cytotoxic effects on stem cells, the ideal concentration remains debated, with proposed ranges between 1.5% and 3% (Galler et al., 2020). Likewise, recommended durations for intracanal material placement differ, with some protocols endorsing a 1-week application of $Ca(OH)_2$ and others supporting the use of antibiotic pastes for 3–4 weeks to achieve more robust disinfection (Zhou et al., 2023). Such procedural variability contributes to inconsistent clinical outcomes and highlights the need for well-designed clinical trials to establish evidence-based, standardized regenerative protocols.

Another challenge in regenerative endodontics concerns the long-term viability and functional fidelity of the regenerated pulp-like tissue. Although numerous cases demonstrate histological evidence of vascularized connective tissue within the canal space, the precise composition of this tissue can vary considerably (Diogenes et al., 2023). In some instances, the regenerated tissue comprises a heterogeneous mix of fibrous tissue, cementum-like deposits, and osteodentin rather than fully functional pulp (Minic et al., 2022). These findings indicate that, while current regenerative approaches can successfully reintroduce living tissue into the canal, the newly formed tissue does not always recapitulate the full biological and physiological characteristics of native pulp. Overcoming this limitation will require advances in biomimetic scaffold design, targeted gene therapy, and more refined growth factor delivery systems to support consistently predictable and functionally appropriate pulp regeneration (Elnawam et al., 2022).

1.6 FUTURE DIRECTIONS IN REGENERATIVE ENDODONTICS

Despite these challenges, regenerative endodontics remains one of the most promising developments in contemporary dental therapeutics, with ongoing research focused on refining existing techniques and broadening clinical applicability. The emergence of synthetic bioengineered scaffolds, including peptide-based hydrogels and nanostructured biomaterials, has demonstrated potential in improving the uniformity and predictability of tissue formation within the root canal (Figure 1.4) (Murray, 2023). Concurrently, CRISPR-mediated gene-editing strategies are being investigated to enhance stem cell viability, proliferation, and lineage commitment, thereby increasing the reliability of regenerative outcomes (Zhou et al., 2023). Looking ahead, the integration of 3D bioprinting technology may enable the

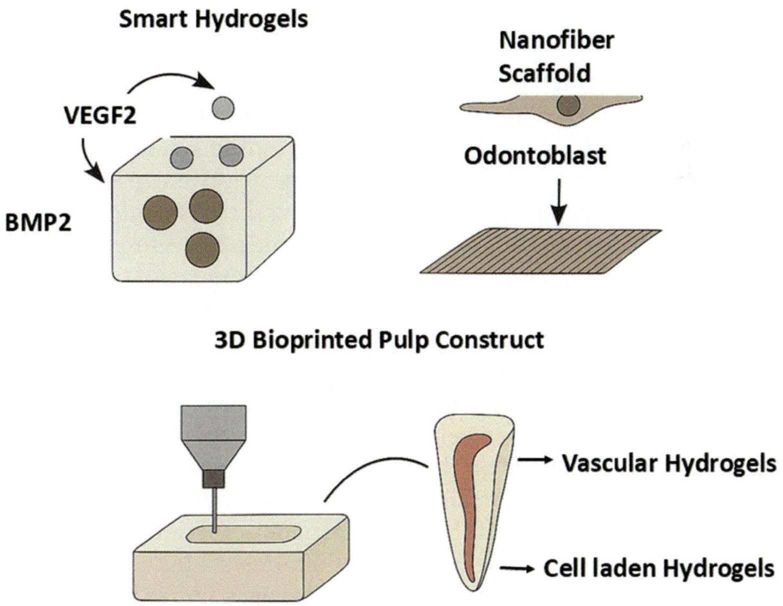

Figure 1.4 Advanced biomaterial and biofabrication strategies for regenerative endodontics. Smart hydrogels enable precise release of growth factors, nanofiber scaffolds provide directional cues for odontoblast-like differentiation, and 3D bioprinting allows the creation of vascularized pulp constructs that match canal anatomy. Together, these technologies enhance the predictability and long-term functionality of regenerative outcomes.

fabrication of patient-specific pulp constructs featuring precisely organized vascular, neural, and odontogenic cell populations, offering unprecedented control over the architecture and functionality of regenerated pulp tissue (Galler et al., 2020). Regenerative endodontics has transformed the management of necrotic immature permanent teeth, and ongoing research aims to refine treatment outcomes, enhance predictability, and expand clinical applications. The focus is shifting toward developing biomimetic scaffold materials, improving disinfection protocols that preserve stem cell viability, and optimizing cell homing techniques to eliminate the need for exogenous stem cell transplantation. These advancements aim to make regenerative endodontics more reliable and accessible while addressing current challenges such as variability in outcomes, inconsistent tissue regeneration, and limitations in treatment standardization.

Another major area of ongoing research involves improving disinfection strategies to ensure effective microbial elimination while preserving the viability of stem cells within the periapical region. Although NaOCl remains the most widely used irrigant due to its strong antimicrobial activity, its cytotoxic effects can impair the ability of residual stem cells to migrate, proliferate, and differentiate, thereby limiting regenerative potential. To address this challenge, recent investigations have evaluated antimicrobial nanoparticles, including silver, chitosan, and graphene oxide-based formulations, which selectively target bacterial cells while exhibiting substantially lower toxicity toward host progenitor cells (Murray, 2023). Additional approaches, such as enzymatic biofilm disruptors and low-energy laser irradiation, have shown promise in destabilizing biofilms and achieving bacterial reduction without compromising the regenerative capacity of SCAP populations (Zhang et al., 2023). Incorporating these emerging antimicrobial modalities into regenerative protocols is anticipated to enhance clinical outcomes by minimizing microbial load while supporting a biologically favorable microenvironment for predictable tissue regeneration.

One of the most transformative advances in regenerative endodontics is the development of cell homing strategies, which aim to recruit endogenous stem and progenitor cells to the site of injury, thereby eliminating the need for exogenous stem cell transplantation. Conventional regenerative approaches rely largely on the passive migration of stem cells from the apical papilla and adjacent periapical tissues into the disinfected root canal. However, the efficiency of this process is variable, especially in cases where severe infection or structural damage has diminished the viability of resident stem cell populations. Cell homing techniques utilize targeted bioactive molecules and chemotactic signals to actively direct stem cells into the canal space, thereby promoting more consistent cellular repopulation and lineage differentiation.

Another promising avenue for enhancing stem cell homing involves the use of bioengineered dentin matrices and biologically preconditioned dentin surfaces. Studies have shown that treating dentin with growth factor-rich formulations, such as EDTA combined with TGF-β, can augment the release of endogenous bioactive molecules sequestered within the dentin matrix, thereby establishing a microenvironment that naturally attracts stem cells and supports their odontogenic differentiation (Galler et al., 2020). This strategy leverages the inherent regenerative potential of dentin while reducing reliance on externally administered biomolecules, offering a biologically efficient approach to improving regenerative outcomes.

In addition to biochemical signaling, gene therapy and molecular engineering are being investigated as strategies to further enhance endogenous cell homing. CRISPR-based gene editing has been explored to upregulate homing-associated receptors on stem cells, thereby increasing their sensitivity and responsiveness to chemotactic cues within the canal microenvironment (Shah and Loghin, 2021). Parallel studies have examined exosome-based therapeutics in which extracellular vesicles derived from stem cells deliver regulatory molecules that promote cell migration, survival, and differentiation. These emerging approaches hold significant potential for improving the precision, efficiency, and reliability of REPs by enabling more targeted recruitment of reparative cell populations.

As regenerative endodontics progresses, the convergence of smart biomaterials, advanced antimicrobial strategies, and precision-driven cell homing technologies will be central to enhancing treatment outcomes. Future directions in the field include the development of programmable scaffolds capable of dynamically interfacing with host tissues, modulating growth factor release, and providing real-time feedback on regenerative progress (Zhou et al., 2023). Moreover, the integration of personalized medicine approaches, such as patient-specific stem cell profiling and customized biomaterial design, may allow regenerative protocols to be tailored to an individual's unique biological characteristics, thereby improving predictability and long-term success.

Future research should also prioritize whole-tooth regeneration, a long-term objective in dental tissue engineering that involves creating bioengineered tooth constructs seeded with autologous stem cells. Although this approach remains experimental, ongoing progress in stem cell differentiation, scaffold design, and vascular integration indicates that the *in situ* generation of a fully functional replacement tooth may eventually become a clinically achievable outcome (Galler et al., 2020).

1.7 CONCLUSION

Regenerative endodontics represents a major advancement in the biologically based management of necrotic teeth, shifting treatment goals from devitalization toward true restoration of pulp-like tissue, vascularity, and continued root development. Although current clinical outcomes are promising, challenges such as variable tissue differentiation, patient-specific responses, and limited long-term evidence highlight the need for protocol standardization and improved biomaterials. Ongoing developments in biomimetic scaffolds, advanced antimicrobial strategies, gene-editing technologies, and targeted cell homing approaches hold considerable potential to enhance the predictability and durability of regenerative outcomes. Emerging tools such as 3D bioprinting and personalized regenerative methods may further expand clinical applicability, offering tailored solutions for pulp tissue loss and trauma. As research continues to translate laboratory advances into clinical practice, regenerative endodontics is poised to redefine modern endodontic therapy, promoting minimally invasive, biologically driven, and patient-centered approaches to long-term tooth preservation.

REFERENCES

Abbass, M. M. S., Al-Haddad, Z. A., Ibrahim, D. H., & Hussein, N. A. (2020). Hydrogels and dentin–pulp complex regeneration: From bench to clinical translation. *Journal of Endodontics*, 46(9), 1296–1311.

American Association of Endodontists. (2021). Guidelines for Regenerative Endodontics. Retrieved from www.aae.org

Bakhtiar, H., Abedi, F., Kharazifard, M. J., & Bagheri, H. (2017). Human pulp responses to partial pulpotomy treatment with enamel matrix derivative: A randomized controlled trial. *Journal of Endodontics*, 43(10), 1619–1625.

Diogenes, A., & Ruparel, N. B. (2017). Regenerative endodontic procedures: Clinical outcomes and future directions. *Journal of Endodontics*, 43(9), S35–S45.

Diogenes, A., Henry, M. A., & Hargreaves, K. M. (2023). Future directions in regenerative endodontics: Harnessing new biomaterials and gene therapy. *Dental Materials*, 39(2), 205–214.

Elnawam, H., Abdelmougod, M., Mobarak, A., Hussein, M., Aboualmakarem, H., Girgis, M., & El Backly, R. (2022). Regenerative endodontics and minimally invasive dentistry: Intertwining paths crossing over into clinical translation. *Frontiers in Bioengineering and Biotechnology*, 10, 837639. doi: 10.3389/fbioe.2022.837639.

Galler, K. M., Widbiller, M., & Buchalla, W. (2020). Advances in the development of bioactive scaffolds for regenerative endodontics. *Frontiers in Bioengineering and Biotechnology*, 8, 605734.

Kim, S. G., Malek, M., Sigurdsson, A., Lin, L. M., & Kahler, B. (2018). Regenerative endodontics: A comprehensive review. *International Endodontic Journal*, 51(12), 1367–1381.

Liu, H., Lu, J., Jiang, Q., Haapasalo, M., Qian, J., Tay, F. R., & Shen, Y. (2022, June). Biomaterial scaffolds for clinical procedures in endodontic regeneration: Biomaterial scaffolds in endodontic regeneration. *Bioactive Materials*, 12, 257–277.

Minic, S., Vital, S., Chaussain, C., Boukpessi, T., & Mangione, F. (2022, Sep 11). Tissue characteristics in endodontic regeneration: A systematic review. *International Journal of Molecular Sciences*, 23(18), 10534. doi: 10.3390/ijms231810534. PMID: 36142446; PMCID: PMC9504778.

Murray, P.E. (2023). Review of guidance for the selection of regenerative endodontics, apexogenesis, apexification, pulpotomy, and other endodontic treatments for immature permanent teeth. *International Endodontic Journal*, 56(Suppl. 2), 188–199. Available from: https://doi.org/10.1111/iej.13809.

Murray, P. E., Garcia-Godoy, F., & Hargreaves, K. M. (2021). Regenerative endodontics: A review of current status and future directions. *Journal of Endodontics*, 44(3), S49–S59.

Shah, N., & Loghin, S. (2021). Regenerative endodontics for mature teeth: Are we ready for clinical translation? *Dental Clinics of North America*, 65(2), 237–252.

Torabinejad, M., & Nosrat, A. (2019). Regenerative endodontics: The role of apical papilla and stem cells. *Dental Research Journal*, 16(3), 167–175.

Zhang, Z., Wang, J., Chen, R., & Zheng, L. (2023). Bioengineered pulp–dentin complex with functional innervation. *Acta Biomaterialia*, 149, 280–299.

Zhou, X., Peng, X., Xu, X., & Yang, G. (2023). Advances in regenerative endodontics: Stem cells and biomaterials for pulp-dentin complex regeneration. *Regenerative Biomaterials*, 10(1), rbm12345.

Chapter 2

3D organoids for regenerative endodontics

2.1 INTRODUCTION

Regenerative endodontics has emerged as a transformative approach in dental medicine, which aims to restore the vitality and function of the dental pulp–dentin complex rather than merely addressing symptoms through traditional methods. This biological restoration is achieved by revitalizing necrotic pulp tissue, promoting the growth of new tissue that closely mimics the original structure and function of the tooth. The advent of three-dimensional (3D) organoid technology has significantly advanced this field by providing biologically relevant models that simulate the *in vivo* environment, thereby enhancing our understanding and application of regenerative endodontic principles.

Central to regenerative endodontics is the utilization of stem cells, which possess the unique ability to differentiate into various cell types necessary for tissue regeneration. Dental pulp stem cells (DPSCs), stem cells from human exfoliated deciduous teeth (SHED), and stem cells from the apical papilla (SCAP) have been extensively studied for their regenerative potential. These cells can differentiate into odontoblast-like cells, contributing to dentin formation and the overall regeneration of the pulp–dentin complex. For instance, SHED have demonstrated the capacity to differentiate into multiple cell lineages, making them a promising candidate for dental tissue engineering (Chang et al., 2020) (Figure 2.1).

The development of the 3D organoid technology has provided a more accurate representation of the *in vivo* environment compared to traditional two-dimensional (2D) cultures. Organoids are self-organizing, multicellular structures that recapitulate key aspects of their tissue of origin, including architecture and function. In regenerative endodontics, dental pulp organoids are generated from stem cells, offering a platform to study the complex interactions within the pulp–dentin complex and to investigate potential therapeutic agents. Recent advancements have demonstrated the potential of microfluidic droplet encapsulation in guiding organoid growth, promoting the recapitulation of parental tumor phenotypes, which could be adapted for dental tissues (W. Zhang et al., 2024).

 DOI: 10.1201/9781003589921-2

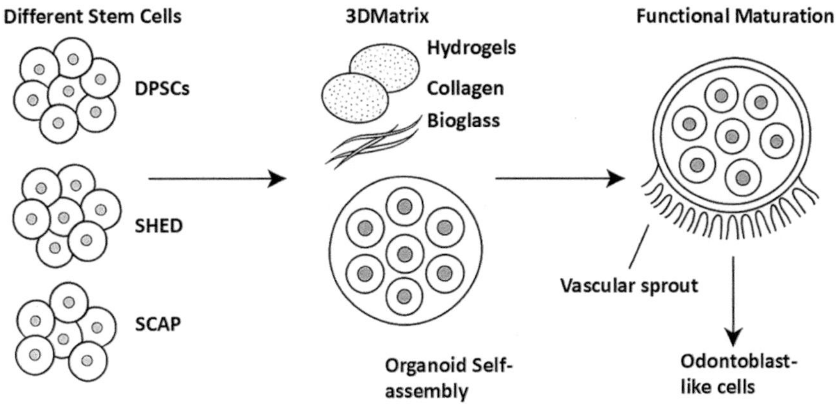

Figure 2.1 Workflow of 3D organoid development for regenerative endodontics. The schematic summarizes the major stages of dental pulp organoid formation, including stem cell isolation, scaffold integration, organoid self-organization, and functional maturation supported by TGF-β1.

The regenerative process is heavily influenced by bioactive molecules and signaling pathways that regulate cell behavior. Transforming growth factor beta 1 (TGF-β1) is a pivotal cytokine involved in odontogenic differentiation and tissue regeneration. Studies have shown that TGF-β1 enhances the regenerative activity of SHED through pathways such as ALK5/Smad2, TAK1, p38, and MEK/ERK signaling (Chang et al., 2020). Additionally, the modification of bioglass materials with TGF-β1-binding peptides has been shown to induce odontogenic differentiation, highlighting the importance of bioactive molecule delivery in regenerative endodontics (Wu et al., 2022).

Besides, the scaffold materials provide the necessary support for cell attachment, proliferation, and differentiation in tissue engineering. The combination of scaffolds with organoids enhances the regenerative potential by creating a conducive microenvironment that mimics the extracellular matrix (ECM) of dental tissues. Natural polymers like collagen and synthetic materials such as bioactive glass have been utilized to fabricate scaffolds that support DPSCs. For example, the use of TGF-β1 binding peptide-modified bioglass has been shown to promote odontogenic differentiation, indicating its potential application in regenerative endodontic therapy (Wu et al., 2022).

2.2 ADVANCES IN 3D CELL CULTURE TECHNIQUES

The advent of 3D cell culture techniques has revolutionized tissue engineering and regenerative medicine, particularly in fields like regenerative endodontics.

2.2.1 Limitations of 2D monolayer cultures

The 2D monolayer cell cultures have long been a cornerstone of biological research, offering a controlled and reproducible environment to study cellular behavior, drug interactions, and basic tissue biology. While these models have provided significant insights into cell biology, their limitations are increasingly apparent in fields such as tissue engineering and regenerative endodontics, where mimicking the complexity of *in vivo* conditions is crucial (Table 2.1). The static and simplistic nature of 2D cultures hinders their ability to accurately model the dynamic and multidimensional environment of living tissues, presenting challenges for translational research and therapeutic development (Figure 2.2).

Table 2.1 Comparison of 2D and 3D cell cultures in regenerative endodontics

Feature	*2D cell culture*	*3D organoid culture*
Tissue architecture	Flat monolayer; lacks tissue complexity	Mimics native tissue structure
Cell–cell interactions	Limited due to 2D growth	Enhanced interactions in 3D arrangement
Gene expression	Altered gene profiles; non-physiological	Closely replicates *in vivo* gene expression
Extracellular matrix (ECM) mimicry	Minimal ECM interaction	Biomimetic ECM-like environment
Cell differentiation	Less accurate differentiation signals	Supports multilineage differentiation
Drug testing relevance	Poor predictive value	More reliable for preclinical studies
Nutrient and oxygen diffusion	Uniform across monolayers	Gradient-based diffusion, similar to tissues

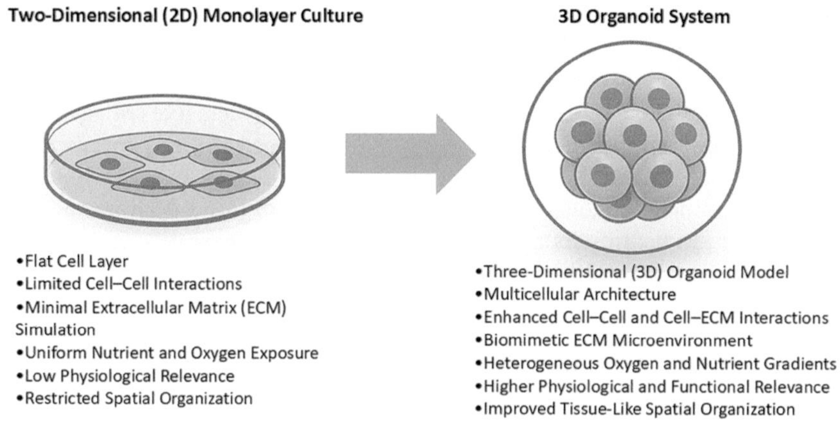

Figure 2.2 Comparison of 2D monolayer cultures and 3D organoid systems. The diagram illustrates structural, biochemical, and functional differences between 2D culture platforms and 3D biomimetic models, highlighting limitations in spatial organization, cell–cell interactions, ECM simulation, and physiological relevance.

2.2.1.1 Lack of spatial organization and tissue architecture

Cells *in vivo* exist in a 3D ECM, which provides structural and biochemical cues essential for proper cellular function. In 2D cultures, the cells grow on a rigid, flat surface, which forces them into unnatural morphologies. For instance, odontoblasts in the dental pulp naturally align along the pulp–dentin interface, a configuration that cannot be replicated in 2D. Further, *in vivo*, cells are polarized, with distinct apical and basal surfaces that interact with their environment. This polarity is lost in 2D cultures, leading to altered cellular behavior. Also, the tissues are composed of diverse cell types interacting dynamically. In the dental pulp, odontoblasts, fibroblasts, endothelial cells, and immune cells coordinate to maintain homeostasis and respond to injury. Such interactions are difficult to model in 2D cultures, where cells are typically cultured in isolation (Edmondson et al., 2014).

2.2.1.2 Altered cellular behavior and gene expression

The artificial and highly simplified architecture of 2D culture systems markedly alters cellular behavior, creating substantial discrepancies between *in vitro* observations and *in vivo* biology. Cells maintained in a 2D environment demonstrate distinct transcriptional profiles relative to those cultured in 3D or native tissue environments. For instance, DPSCs grown in a 2D environment exhibit diminished expression of odontogenic markers, which in turn compromises their differentiation capacity (Duval et al., 2017). Cellular signaling is also profoundly regulated by the surrounding microenvironment, and the lack of an ECM-like context in 2D settings disrupts critical pathways governing adhesion, proliferation, and lineage. Consequently, findings derived from 2D systems often fail to translate reliably to physiologically relevant or clinical contexts.

2.2.1.3 Poor simulation of the extracellular microenvironment

In vivo, the ECM functions as a dynamic and bioactive scaffold that modulates cellular behavior through integrated mechanical and biochemical cues. In contrast, 2D culture substrates lack the native stiffness, elasticity, and topographical complexity characteristic of the ECM. These biophysical properties are essential regulators of odontoblast differentiation and dentinogenesis, and their absence in 2D systems leads to incomplete recapitulation of physiological tissue development. Also, in living tissues, gradients of nutrients, oxygen, and signaling molecules guide cellular behavior. In 2D settings, the uniform exposure to culture media eliminates these gradients, limiting the ability to study phenomena such as hypoxia-induced angiogenesis (Huang et al., 2010).

2.2.1.4 Limited cell–cell and cell–ECM interactions

Cell–environment interactions are fundamental to maintaining tissue homeostasis, facilitating repair, and driving regenerative processes. In 2D cultures, cells interact with adjacent cells and extracellular signals primarily along a single plane, lacking the multidirectional and spatially integrated communication that occurs within 3D tissues. This geometric limitation reduces the physiological relevance of key biological events such as immune cell recruitment, vascular network formation, and angiogenic signaling. As a result, 2D systems provide an incomplete model for investigating immune dynamics and angiogenesis in dental pulp regeneration.

2.2.1.5 Static culture conditions

In vivo, tissues are exposed to dynamic biophysical conditions, including fluid flow, mechanical loading, and spatial nutrient gradients, all of which profoundly influence cellular proliferation, differentiation, and functional maturation. The 2D culture systems, however, rely on static media environments that do not recapitulate the fluid dynamics essential for efficient nutrient transport and metabolic waste clearance. Shear forces generated by physiological fluid flow, such as blood perfusion, are key regulators of vascular development and angiogenesis. Within the dental pulp, these hemodynamic cues critically govern the formation and maturation of new blood vessels, an indispensable component of successful regenerative outcomes.

2.2.1.6 Limited predictive value for translational research

The simplified architecture of 2D culture systems restricts their capacity to model complex biological processes, thereby limiting their predictive value for translational and clinical applications. In drug screening, for example, compounds that demonstrate efficacy in 2D models frequently fail during clinical evaluation because these systems do not reproduce the physiologically relevant microenvironment required for accurate assessment of the drug response. Moreover, the static and planar nature of 2D cultures precludes the formation of 3D tissue-like constructs capable of integrating with native structures, a fundamental requirement in regenerative endodontics (Tibbitt and Anseth, 2009).

2.2.1.7 Challenges in modeling inflammation and immune responses

The dental pulp is a highly vascularized tissue enriched with diverse immune cell populations that orchestrate inflammation, host defense, and tissue repair. In 2D culture systems, the absence of immune components or the limited capacity to co-culture multiple cell types severely restricts the ability to model these processes. As a result, key inflammatory events relevant to conditions such as pulpitis cannot be accurately reproduced. Likewise, complex and dynamic interactions among immune cells, stem cells, and endothelial cells that drive coordinated tissue repair and regeneration cannot be recapitulated in 2D environments, underscoring their limitations for studying pulp biology and regenerative mechanisms.

2.3 DEVELOPMENT AND APPLICATION OF 3D MODELS

The advent of 3D cell culture systems has markedly advanced tissue engineering and regenerative medicine by providing biologically sophisticated platforms for investigating cellular behavior and tissue formation. In regenerative endodontics, 3D culture models more accurately recapitulate the complex architecture and functional dynamics of the pulp–dentin complex, thereby enabling detailed mechanistic studies and facilitating the development of targeted therapeutic strategies. By overcoming the inherent limitations of traditional 2D monolayer cultures, these models establish a physiologically relevant microenvironment that more closely aligns *in vitro* findings with *in vivo* biology, effectively narrowing the translational gap between experimental research and clinical application.

2.3.1 Evolution of 3D cell culture models

The emergence of 3D culture models is rooted in the need to transcend the static, oversimplified conditions inherent to 2D systems. Progress in biomaterials engineering, microfabrication technologies, and stem cell biology has propelled the development of diverse 3D platforms, including multicellular spheroids, organoids, hydrogel-based scaffolds, and bioprinted constructs. These systems reproduce the structural, biochemical, and mechanical properties of native tissues, providing advanced tools for studying development, disease, and regeneration. In the next section, the different 3D systems are introduced.

A. Spheroid Cultures: Among the earliest and most widely used 3D systems are spherical aggregates of cells formed under non-adherent culture conditions. By promoting natural cell–cell and cell–matrix interactions, spheroids generate oxygen, nutrient, and signaling gradients reminiscent of *in vivo* tissues. This creates a microenvironment that enhances lineage commitment and functional maturation. In regenerative endodontics, spheroids derived from DPSCs have shown superior odontogenic differentiation, ECM deposition, and pro-angiogenic activity relative to monolayers. For instance, Yamamoto et al. (2020) demonstrated that DPSC spheroids embedded in ECM mimetic hydrogels generated dentin-like structures with markedly improved structural integrity. Building upon the strengths of spheroids, more complex 3D systems have been developed to further recapitulate tissue organization.

B. Organoids: Organoids represent a more advanced level of 3D biomimicry, forming through the self-organization of stem cells into multicellular structures that recapitulate key architectural and functional features of native tissues. Dental pulp organoids recreate the spatial arrangement of odontoblasts, fibroblasts, and endothelial cells, enabling detailed investigations of physiological processes, disease mechanisms, and therapeutic responses. Recent innovations have generated vascularized dental pulp organoids, which exhibit enhanced nutrient exchange, viability, and longevity *in vitro* (Li and Kishen, 2023). While organoids offer improved complexity compared with spheroids, their microenvironments can be further refined using engineered ECMs, such as hydrogels.
C. Hydrogel-Based Scaffolds: Hydrogel-based scaffolds serve as highly versatile 3D matrices that closely emulate the biochemical and biophysical properties of the native ECM. Their tunable stiffness, porosity, and degradability allow for precise modulation of cell behavior, while their capacity to incorporate bioactive molecules and multiple cell types enables the formation of tissue-specific constructs. Injectable hydrogels loaded with DPSCs and angiogenic factors, such as vascular endothelial growth factor (VEGF), have successfully generated pulp-like tissues containing organized vasculature and polarized odontoblast layers (Huang et al., 2010). Although hydrogels create supportive ECM-like environments, recent advancements aim to achieve even greater spatial precision through additive manufacturing techniques.
D. 3D Bioprinting: 3D bioprinting represents the most customizable and structurally precise platform among current 3D culture technologies. This approach fabricates tissue constructs in a layer-by-layer manner using bioinks composed of cells, biomaterials, and signaling molecules, allowing for accurate control over the spatial architecture. Such precision is essential for replicating the complex anatomy of the pulp–dentin interface. Zhao et al. (2024) demonstrated the successful bioprinting of pulp–dentin-like constructs containing aligned odontoblast-like cells and integrated vascular networks, validating the potential of bioprinting for constructing functional tissues suitable for translational regenerative applications.

2.4 APPLICATIONS OF 3D ORGANOIDS IN REGENERATIVE ENDODONTICS

In regenerative endodontics, accurately modeling the dynamic cellular and molecular interactions that govern pulpal and periapical biology is essential for developing effective therapeutic interventions. 3D organoids, which closely recapitulate the architectural complexity and cellular heterogeneity of native dental tissues, have emerged as a powerful platform for investigating these processes. By reproducing key features of the *in vivo* microenvironment, organoid systems enable detailed exploration of tissue homeostasis, inflammatory responses, and repair mechanisms, thereby providing critical insights into the pathophysiology of endodontic diseases and the regenerative potential of new treatment approaches.

2.4.1 Pulpal tissue dynamics

The dental pulp is a specialized soft connective tissue enclosed within the rigid dentin, and it is indispensable for maintaining tooth vitality. Its complex anatomy, characterized by dense vascularization and extensive innervation, supports essential functions including odontogenesis, immune surveillance, and sensory transduction. The coordinated activity of its heterogeneous cellular populations underpins tissue homeostasis, orchestrates inflammatory responses, and drives regenerative processes following injury. The development of 3D organoid systems has transformed the study of pulpal biology by offering highly biomimetic models that replicate key aspects of the native microenvironment. These organoids enable sophisticated analyses of cellular dynamics, molecular signaling pathways, and therapeutic responses, thereby advancing research and innovation in regenerative endodontics.

2.4.2 Cellular composition and function

The dental pulp comprises multiple specialized cell types, each contributing to its structural organization and functional resilience. The coordinated interactions among odontoblasts, fibroblasts, endothelial cells, pericytes, and immune cells form the core of pulpal tissue dynamics, influencing homeostasis, defense, and regeneration (Figure 2.3). 3D organoid systems successfully recapitulate this cellular heterogeneity, offering a physiologically relevant platform for investigating normal tissue physiology and the mechanisms underlying disease. The specific cell types within the dental pulp and their respective functional roles are examined in detail in the following section.

2.4.2.1 Odontoblasts

Odontoblasts, the highly specialized cells lining the periphery of the pulp chamber, play a central role in dentinogenesis. These post-mitotic cells synthesize primary dentin during tooth development and continue to form secondary dentin throughout life. Upon exposure to pathological stimuli such as carious insult or mechanical trauma, odontoblasts initiate the production of tertiary dentin to safeguard the underlying pulp. Their polarized

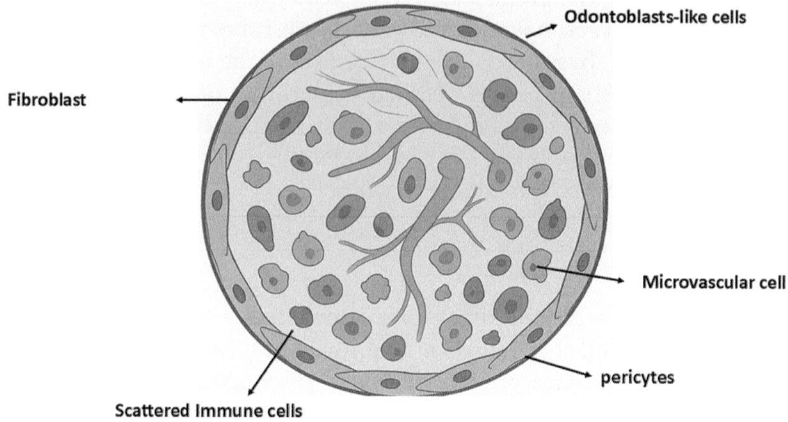

Figure 2.3 Cellular organization within dental pulp organoids. The schematic depicts major cell populations present in pulp organoids, including odontoblast-like cells, fibroblasts, endothelial cells, pericytes, and resident immune cells, arranged in a biomimetic microarchitecture that mirrors native pulp tissue.

morphology, characterized by an apical process extending into the dentinal tubules, enables the detection of mechanical, thermal, and chemical cues from the external environment. These stimuli activate intracellular pathways that drive the secretion of dentin matrix components, including collagen, dentin sialophosphoprotein (DSPP), and dentin matrix protein-1 (DMP-1).

In organoid-based models, odontoblast-like cells retain this intrinsic polarity and deposit dentin-like matrix, thereby closely mimicking their *in vivo* function (Kim et al., 2021). Such biomimetic systems allow detailed examination of odontoblast behavior under both physiological and pathological conditions. They also provide a controlled environment for studying odontoblast responses to bacterial invasion, inflammatory mediators, bioactive materials, and restorative procedures, offering valuable insights that inform the development of improved regenerative and therapeutic strategies.

2.4.2.2 *Fibroblasts*

Fibroblasts are the most abundant cellular population within the dental pulp and play a pivotal role in maintaining ECM homeostasis and modulating the immune activity. As key regulators of ECM remodeling, fibroblasts synthesize and degrade structural components such as collagen, fibronectin, and proteoglycans. They orchestrate ECM turnover through the secretion of matrix metalloproteinases and their endogenous inhibitors, thereby preserving a dynamic balance between matrix formation and degradation. In organoid systems, the inclusion of fibroblasts recreates the ECM-rich milieu characteristic of native pulp tissue, offering a robust platform to investigate fibroblast-mediated interactions with odontoblasts, endothelial cells, and immune cells. These models have demonstrated that fibroblasts not only support odontoblast differentiation by modulating matrix composition and mechanical signals but also contribute to coordinated immune responses during injury, underscoring their central role in pulpal repair and regeneration.

2.4.2.3 *Endothelial cells and pericytes*

The vascular network of the dental pulp is fundamental to tissue vitality, providing continuous nutrient delivery, metabolic waste removal, and coordinated immune cell trafficking. Endothelial cells, which line the interior surface of blood vessels, regulate vascular permeability, angiogenic signaling, and leukocyte migration. In response to injury, these cells upregulate pro-angiogenic mediators such as VEGF, driving the formation of new microvessels to reestablish tissue perfusion. Pericytes, which sheath endothelial cells along the microvasculature, serve essential stabilizing functions by regulating vascular tone, controlling permeability, and guiding vessel maturation. Through their combined roles in angiogenesis and microvascular maintenance, endothelial cells and pericytes are central to pulpal homeostasis.

Incorporating both cell types into 3D organoid systems has enabled the generation of vascularized dental pulp models that closely mimic the native microcirculatory architecture. These advanced biomimetic constructs support detailed investigation of vascular processes, including VEGF-driven angiogenesis, endothelial–pericyte interactions, and the impact of vascular remodeling on tissue repair and regeneration (Yamamoto et al., 2020). Such models provide critical mechanistic insights into pulp regeneration and inform the development of more effective regenerative endodontic therapies.

2.4.2.4 *Immune cells*

The dental pulp harbors a diverse population of immune cells, including macrophages, dendritic cells, and mast cells, which constitute the primary defense system against invading pathogens. These cells continuously survey the microenvironment for signs of microbial intrusion or tissue injury and initiate an immediate inflammatory response when such signals are detected. Macrophages play a central role by phagocytosing pathogens and releasing pro-inflammatory cytokines such as interleukin 1 beta and tumor necrosis factor alpha, which recruit additional immune cells to the affected site. The capacity to examine macrophage-mediated cytokine signaling and immune cell crosstalk within 3D organoid systems offers valuable insights into their contributions to inflammation modulation and tissue repair.

The dental pulp is routinely subjected to various injuries, including microbial invasion, mechanical trauma, and restorative interventions, all of which trigger a coordinated cascade of cellular and molecular responses to maintain tissue integrity. Injury activates resident immune cells and promotes the recruitment of circulating leukocytes into the pulp, a process driven by inflammatory mediators such as interleukin 6 and tumor necrosis factor alpha. These cytokines increase vascular permeability, enabling neutrophils, macrophages, and lymphocytes to migrate into the injured tissue and participate in host defense.

3D organoid models provide a controlled and physiologically relevant environment for replicating and studying these inflammatory processes. By enabling dynamic interactions among immune cells, odontoblasts, fibroblasts, and endothelial cells, organoids facilitate a detailed understanding of how inflammation is coordinated and resolved during pulp injury and how these mechanisms contribute to subsequent tissue regeneration.

2.5 ODONTOBLAST SURVIVAL AND REPARATIVE FUNCTION

Understanding how odontoblasts survive and function following injury is fundamental to regenerative endodontics as these cells form the first defensive and reparative barrier within the pulp. Odontoblasts are highly specialized cells responsible for dentinogenesis and maintaining the structural integrity of the pulp–dentin interface. When exposed to insults such as caries, trauma, or restorative procedures, surviving odontoblasts initiate the synthesis of tertiary dentin, sealing damaged areas and restoring pulpal protection. This reparative process is mediated by the upregulation of genes encoding key dentin matrix proteins, including DSPP and DMP-1.

3D organoid systems offer a powerful platform to study odontoblast behavior under controlled inflammatory or stress conditions. Within these models, researchers can examine how odontoblasts respond to toll-like receptor activation, the presence of bacterial components, or exposure to bioactive molecules such as transforming growth factor beta 1. These insights are critical for characterizing odontoblast mediated repair and for developing therapeutic strategies that enhance tertiary dentin formation. A comprehensive understanding of odontoblast responses requires integration with the broader biological environment of the periapical region, where tissue dynamics significantly influence pulpal survival, inflammation, and regeneration (Figure 2.4).

2.5.1 Periapical tissue dynamics

The periapical region, located at the root apex, is a biologically active environment that contributes to tooth stability, immune defense, and regenerative potential. Its structural and functional complexity arises from the coordinated activity of fibroblasts, osteoblasts, osteoclasts, immune cells,

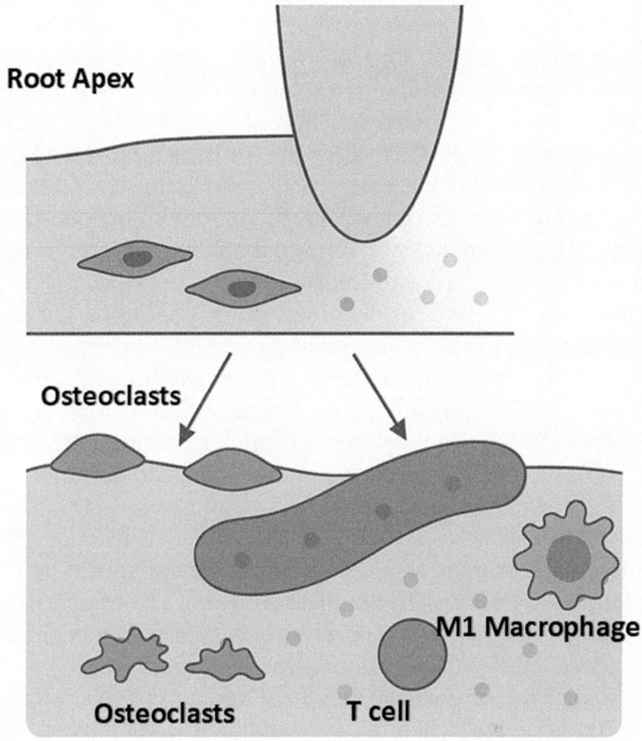

Figure 2.4 Biomimetic periapical organoid model. The diagram integrates osteoblasts, osteoclasts, fibroblasts, vascular elements, and immune cells to illustrate how organoid systems recreate the dynamic microenvironment of the periapical region, enabling controlled study of inflammation, bone remodeling, and regenerative processes.

vascular networks, and neural components. These cellular interactions maintain homeostasis under physiological conditions and orchestrate adaptive responses following injury. Pathological stimuli such as microbial invasion or trauma disrupt these dynamics, leading to inflammatory changes, bone remodeling, and potential tooth loss. Advances in three-dimensional organoid technologies now enable the replication of periapical microenvironments with high fidelity, allowing researchers to study cellular interactions, molecular signaling, and therapeutic responses in physiologically relevant systems.

2.5.1.1 Cellular composition of periapical tissue

A. Fibroblasts: Fibroblasts form the dominant stromal population within the periodontal ligament and periapical tissues. They maintain structural integrity by synthesizing collagen types I and III, fibronectin, and proteoglycans, which confer mechanical resilience and flexibility. By producing matrix metalloproteinases and tissue inhibitors of metalloproteinases, fibroblasts regulate extracellular matrix turnover, enabling tissue adaptation and repair (Duka et al., 2019). During inflammation, fibroblasts respond to cytokines such as IL-1β and TNF-α by secreting prostaglandins and chemokines that amplify leukocyte recruitment and influence osteoclast activation, thereby contributing indirectly to bone resorption (Huang et al., 2024). Three-dimensional organoid platforms that integrate fibroblasts enable detailed examination of their crosstalk with osteoblasts, endothelial cells, and resident immune populations. These multicellular systems replicate the dynamic microenvironment of inflamed periapical tissues and provide mechanistic insights into how fibroblasts regulate ECM remodeling, modulate inflammatory signaling, and contribute to the progression of apical periodontitis (Kim et al., 2021).

B. Osteoblasts and Osteoclasts: Bone remodeling in the periapical region depends on the coupled actions of osteoblasts and osteoclasts. Osteoblasts, derived from mesenchymal stem cells, are responsible for producing bone matrix proteins including collagen type I, osteopontin, and osteocalcin. Their differentiation and mineralizing activity are governed by signaling pathways such as bone morphogenetic protein (BMP) and Wnt/β-catenin (Huang et al., 2024).

   Osteoclasts, originating from the monocyte–macrophage lineage, mediate bone resorption by secreting acidic compounds and proteolytic enzymes including tartrate-resistant acid phosphatase. RANKL is essential for osteoclast maturation, and its upregulation during chronic inflammation drives the bone resorption seen in apical periodontitis (Duka et al., 2019). Organoid platforms incorporating both osteoblasts and osteoclasts permit controlled modeling of bone remodeling dynamics. These systems allow researchers to understand the role of pro-inflammatory cytokines such as TNF-α and IL-6 influence osteoclastogenesis and bone turnover under pathological conditions (Zhao et al., 2024).

C. Immune Cells: Immune cells orchestrate the initiation, amplification, and resolution of periapical inflammation. Macrophages play a dual role, during early inflammation, they release IL-1β, TNF-α, and IL-6 to recruit neutrophils and lymphocytes, while in later stages, they transition into an anti-inflammatory phenotype that produces IL-10 and TGF-β to support tissue repair (Kim et al., 2021). Neutrophils act as first responders, generating reactive oxygen species and antimicrobial peptides to eliminate pathogens. Lymphocytes, particularly T cells, contribute to antigen-specific adaptive immune responses and regulate chronic inflammation. Three-dimensional organoid models enable co-culture of immune cells with fibroblasts and osteoblasts, providing a more accurate representation of the periapical microenvironment. These models have been instrumental in examining leukocyte recruitment, macrophage polarization, and immune-mediated modulation of bone remodeling in apical periodontitis (Duka et al., 2019).

D. Vascular and Neural Networks: Vascularization and innervation are essential for maintaining periapical tissue vitality and facilitating regeneration. Endothelial cells regulate vascular permeability and drive angiogenesis through VEGF-mediated signaling, ensuring sufficient oxygen and nutrient delivery during tissue repair (Zhao et al., 2024). Neural elements contribute not only to nociception but also to inflammatory modulation. Neuropeptides such as substance P and calcitonin gene-related peptide influence immune cell activation and vascular responses, demonstrating the close functional integration of neural and vascular networks (Kim et al., 2021). Organoid models incorporating endothelial cells successfully recreate angiogenic processes and enable the study of osteoblast–endothelial interactions during bone regeneration. Emerging systems integrating neural crest-derived cells further allow examination of neural regulation of periapical dynamics (Huang et al., 2024).

2.5.1.2 *Inflammatory responses in periapical tissue*

Inflammation is the hallmark of periapical pathologies, particularly apical periodontitis, which arises from microbial invasion of the root canal system. Recognition of microbial antigens by toll-like receptors on immune cells activates a cytokine cascade involving IL-1β, TNF-α, and IL-6. These cytokines promote neutrophil recruitment, activate macrophages, and enhance osteoclast differentiation through RANKL signaling, ultimately contributing to bone resorption (Duka et al., 2019). Three-dimensional organoid systems allow the controlled introduction of microbial components or inflammatory mediators, enabling researchers to dissect immune activation pathways and evaluate anti-inflammatory regenerative therapies (Zhao et al., 2024).

2.6 DEVELOPMENT OF DENTAL PULP ORGANOIDS

Dental pulp organoids are three-dimensional constructs engineered to reproduce the intricate architecture and functional characteristics of native dental pulp tissue. They represent an emerging class of biomimetic models that enable precise investigation of pulpal development, disease mechanisms, and regenerative strategies. The fabrication of dental pulp organoids relies on integrating stem cell biology, scaffold engineering, and advanced biofabrication methodologies, each contributing to the reconstruction of a microenvironment that closely approximates in vivo conditions. The foundation of dental pulp organoid formation lies in the careful selection and preparation of stem cells. Dental pulp stem cells are widely used owing to their multipotent differentiation capacity into odontoblasts, osteoblasts, neural-like cells, and other lineages relevant to pulp regeneration. Isolation of DPSCs typically involves the extraction of pulp tissue from human teeth, enzymatic digestion, and expansion in defined culture media that maintain cellular viability, proliferation, and stemness. The purity and biological quality of these cells are crucial, as they constitute the primary cellular component driving the organoid's structural and functional maturation.

2.6.1 Scaffold design and biomaterials

Scaffolds form a three-dimensional framework that supports cellular attachment, proliferation, and differentiation within organoids, and their design is pivotal for replicating the extracellular matrix of natural pulp tissue. Biomaterials used in scaffold fabrication must emulate the biochemical signals and mechanical characteristics of native ECM. Natural polymers such as collagen, gelatin, and hyaluronic acid are commonly used due to their inherent biocompatibility and resemblance to pulpal ECM components. Synthetic materials including poly (lactic-co-glycolic acid) (PLGA) and polyethylene glycol (PEG) provide tunable mechanical properties and controlled degradation profiles, enabling customization to experimental needs (Table 2.2).

Advances in fabrication technologies such as electrospinning and 3D bioprinting allow the generation of scaffolds with defined fiber orientation, porosity, and spatial architecture, enhancing their ability to reproduce the microstructural organization of the dental pulp.

Table 2.2 Types of scaffolds used in 3D organoid culture for endodontics

Scaffold type	*Composition*	*Function in 3D Organoids*	*Advantages*
Hydrogel-based scaffolds	Natural/synthetic polymers (e.g., collagen and gelatin)	Mimics ECM and supports cell attachment	High biocompatibility and tunable stiffness
Bioactive glass scaffolds	Silica-based bioactive materials	Stimulates odontoblast differentiation	Enhances mineralization and provides long-term stability
Nanofiber scaffolds	Electrospun polymer fibers	Provides high surface area for cell growth	Mimics ECM structure and improves cellular organization
3D-bioprinted scaffolds	Layer-by-layer deposition of biomaterials	Enables precise spatial control over cell placement	Customizable; allows vascularization

2.6.2 Biofabrication techniques

The assembly of stem cells and scaffolds into functional organoids requires precise biofabrication strategies. Spheroid culture methods allow DPSCs to self-aggregate into three-dimensional clusters, promoting cell–cell communication and physiological organization. More sophisticated systems, such as microfluidic platforms, introduce tightly controlled microenvironments for cell encapsulation, patterning, and differentiation. Microfluidic droplet-based encapsulation, for example, has been shown to enhance organoid organization and phenotypic fidelity in tumor models (W. Zhang et al., 2024), and the same principles can be adapted to dental pulp organoid engineering. These systems enable precise modulation of nutrient gradients, cell distribution, and shear stress, thereby improving reproducibility and functional maturation of organoids.

2.6.3 Optimization of culture conditions

Establishing an optimal culture environment is critical for supporting organoid growth, differentiation, and long-term maintenance. Specialized media formulations supplemented with growth factors, such as transforming growth factor beta and BMPs, direct DPSCs toward odontogenic and other lineage-specific pathways. Regulation of intracellular signaling cascades is equally essential; for instance, TGF-β1 has been shown to modulate regenerative activity in SHED cells through ALK5/Smad2, TAK1, p38, and MEK/ERK pathways (Chang et al., 2020). Additionally, physiologically relevant oxygen tension, mechanical signals, and extracellular calcium levels can further enhance cellular differentiation, matrix secretion, and overall tissue organization. These parameters collectively guide the maturation and functional fidelity of dental pulp organoids.

2.6.4 Characterization and validation

A comprehensive characterization is required to confirm that organoids accurately replicate the composition and functionality of native dental pulp. Histological and immunohistochemical analyses assess tissue organization, cellular distribution, and expression of odontogenic markers such as DSPP, DMP-1, and collagen type I. Functional validation may include assessing responses to inflammatory stimuli, mechanical stress, or biomaterial exposure. For instance, studies examining the expression of cytokines and defensins in dental pulp tissues (Ayoub et al., 2017) provide reference profiles for evaluating immune competence within organoids. Such multimodal characterization ensures that the constructed organoid model is robust, reproducible, and suitable for downstream experimental applications.

Table 2.3 Applications of 3D organoids in regenerative endodontics

Application	*Description*	*Example*
Pulp regeneration	Restores pulp-like tissue inside necrotic teeth	DPSC-derived organoids forming pulp-like structures
Drug testing and toxicity studies	Evaluates biomaterial and drug interactions	Testing fluoride-based agents on pulp organoids
Modeling inflammation and immune responses	Simulates pulpal infections and healing mechanisms	Studying immune cell activity in periapical organoids
Biomaterial evaluation	Tests scaffolds for endodontic tissue engineering	Assessment of bioactive glasses for dentin formation
Disease modeling	Investigates pathological changes in dental tissues	Modeling of apical periodontitis using patient-derived cells

2.6.5 Applications in regenerative dentistry

Dental pulp organoids hold considerable promise in regenerative dentistry and translational research. They provide versatile platforms for testing bioactive materials, evaluating cellular responses to therapeutic agents, and modeling regenerative outcomes (Table 2.3). Injectable tissue-specific hydrogel systems developed for pulp–dentin regeneration (Han et al., 2024) are assessed within organoids to determine their ability to support cell encapsulation, vascularization, and matrix deposition before progressing to *in vivo* studies. Organoids also enable systematic investigation of conditioning agents and biological factors that influence DPSC behavior, thereby facilitating optimization of clinical protocols for pulp repair and regeneration (Sadaghiani et al., 2016). Through these applications, dental pulp organoids are emerging as powerful tools that bridge fundamental biology with therapeutic innovation.

2.7 PULP REGENERATION AND ROOT DEVELOPMENT

Dental pulp organoids hold significant promise in regenerative dentistry and translational research, providing biologically robust platforms for evaluating biomaterials, therapeutic interventions, and mechanisms underlying pulp regeneration. Their 3D organization allows precise interrogation of how bioactive materials influence cellular behavior, lineage commitment, and matrix formation within a physiologically relevant microenvironment. For example, injectable tissue-specific hydrogel systems developed for pulp–dentin regeneration (Han et al., 2024) can be evaluated in organoid models to determine their effectiveness in supporting DPSC encapsulation, promoting vascular network formation, and enhancing ECM deposition before advancing to *in vivo* studies. In addition, organoids offer a controlled setting for systematically investigating conditioning agents and molecular signals that modulate DPSC proliferation, differentiation, and immunomodulatory functions, thereby informing the optimization of clinical protocols for pulp repair and regeneration (Sadaghiani et al., 2016).

2.8 3D ORGANOIDS FOR DENTAL PULP REGENERATION

The application of 3D organoid systems in pulp regeneration has expanded over the past decade, driven by their ability to recapitulate the biological complexity of native pulp tissue. Organoids derived from DPSCs have been particularly valuable in reconstructing the dental pulp microenvironment, enabling detailed investigations of cellular behavior, lineage specification, and tissue–tissue interactions under physiologically relevant conditions. A landmark study by Han et al. (2024) exemplifies the translational potential of these systems. They developed an injectable, tissue-specific hydrogel designed for pulp–dentin regeneration and used it as a bioactive matrix for DPSC encapsulation. The collagen-based hydrogel featured tunable mechanical properties that differentially influenced DPSC fate. Softer hydrogels (3 mg/mL) enhanced endothelial differentiation, supporting the development of vascular networks essential for pulp vitality. In contrast, stiffer hydrogels (10 mg/mL) promoted odontogenic differentiation, leading to the deposition of dentin-like matrix.

When implanted *in vivo*, these hydrogel constructs successfully generated functional pulp–dentin complexes, demonstrating organized vasculature, odontoblast-like cell alignment, and mineralized tissue formation. Collectively, these findings highlight the capacity of DPSC organoid systems to guide lineage-specific regeneration and underscore the potential of injectable hydrogels as minimally invasive, clinically scalable platforms for dental pulp therapy (Han et al., 2024).

2.9 ROLE OF STEM CELL PLASTICITY IN PULP AND ROOT REGENERATION

The inherent plasticity of dental stem cells is a key determinant of their regenerative potential, enabling them to respond dynamically to developmental signals, injury, and environmental changes. Recent work by Krivanek et al. (2023) elucidated the fluidity of epithelial and mesenchymal stem cell niches within the dental pulp, revealing that these niches undergo continuous and reversible cellular transitions governed by extracellular signals and intrinsic molecular programs. This study underscored how such plasticity can be strategically harnessed in conjunction with 3D organoid systems to promote coordinated regeneration of both pulp and root tissues. Importantly, exploiting the adaptive behavior of these stem cell populations offers opportunities to enhance tissue integration, functional restoration, and long-term stability of regenerated pulp–dentin complexes in clinical applications.

2.10 ENGINEERING APPROACHES IN ORGANOID DEVELOPMENT FOR DENTAL APPLICATIONS

Engineering advancements have played a pivotal role in enhancing the reproducibility, scalability, and functional precision of 3D organoid systems for dental applications. Zhang et al. (2022) highlighted how the integration of chemical, mechanical, and computational approaches can be used to fine-tune organoid development, enabling more accurate control over organoid morphology, cellular composition, and differentiation trajectories. Such approaches are highly relevant to dental pulp and root regeneration, where precise orchestration of cell fate and spatial organization is essential (Figure 2.5). Microfluidic technologies, for example, have enabled the incorporation of controlled nutrient flow, oxygen gradients, and mechanical signals into organoid culture systems. These conditions simulate aspects of the native dental pulp environment, particularly vascular perfusion and metabolic exchange, which are critical for tissue maturation and long-term viability. Furthermore, computational modeling and bioinformatics tools have facilitated the prediction and optimization of growth factor combinations, improving the efficiency of odontogenic and angiogenic differentiation within organoid constructs. Together, these engineering innovations significantly strengthen the translational applicability of dental organoids and accelerate the development of next-generation regenerative strategies.

2.11 TRANSLATIONAL POTENTIAL AND CLINICAL IMPLICATIONS

The translational potential of 3D organoid technology in dentistry is extensive, extending well beyond its applications in tissue regeneration. Dental pulp organoids serve as sophisticated *in vitro* platforms for testing novel biomaterials, optimizing drug delivery systems, and elucidating the molecular mechanisms underlying pulpal and periapical diseases. Their ability to recapitulate key features of native tissue architecture and function makes them highly valuable for preclinical evaluation of therapeutic strategies. In a clinical context, organoid-based approaches have the capacity to transform the management of pulp pathologies by enabling personalized regenerative therapies. For example, autologous DPSCs can be expanded and assembled

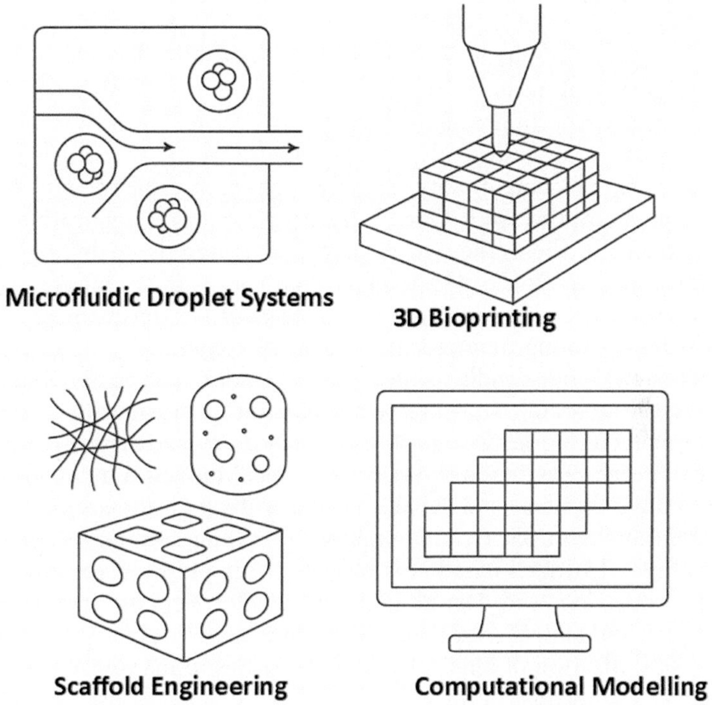

Figure 2.5 Engineering strategies used to enhance dental pulp organoid development. The figure integrates microfluidic droplet systems, 3D bioprinting, scaffold fabrication techniques, and computational modeling workflows that collectively optimize organoid morphology, nutrient exchange, and lineage-specific differentiation.

into patient-specific organoids, which can then be implanted to restore damaged pulp tissue. This strategy not only reduces the risk of immune rejection but also enhances the biological compatibility and long-term functionality of regenerated tissues, positioning organoid technology as a promising next-generation modality for precision endodontic care.

2.12 ORGANOIDS FOR DRUG TESTING AND TOXICITY STUDIES

Over the past decade, the emergence of 3D organoid technologies has transformed drug testing and toxicity assessment across biomedical fields. Traditional 2D cultures and animal models frequently fail to capture the cellular heterogeneity, biomechanical signals, and microenvironmental complexity characteristic of human tissues, resulting in limited predictive value. In contrast, organoids provide architecturally and functionally sophisticated tissue mimetics, making them especially valuable in dentistry, where biomaterial development and drug evaluation require precise modeling of oral tissue interactions. Organoids derived from oral and dental stem cells offer physiologically relevant platforms for assessing the safety, efficacy, and biocompatibility, thereby informing the design of next-generation dental therapies. One of the most important applications of oral organoids lies in the evaluation of dental biomaterials, including composites, adhesives, scaffolds, and implant coatings. Unlike conventional testing systems, organoids simulate the biochemical and mechanical milieu of oral tissues, enabling nuanced assessment of material–tissue interactions. Dental materials must endure salivary enzymes, fluctuating pH, masticatory forces, and microbial exposure while remaining biologically compatible; however, predicting adverse responses such as cytotoxicity or inflammation remains challenging in standard preclinical models. Organoids derived from gingival fibroblasts or DPSCs provide a biologically accurate context for evaluating cytotoxicity, inflammatory signaling, and ECM remodeling. For example, hydrogel-based scaffolds used for pulp regeneration exhibit stiffness-dependent and degradation-dependent effects on odontoblast differentiation and matrix secretion. Testing such scaffolds in organoid cultures enables optimization of biomechanical properties to maximize regenerative outcomes. The evaluation of metallic and nanoparticle-based biomaterials has also been significantly advanced by organoid models. Titanium dioxide and silver nanoparticles (AgNPs), widely incorporated into dental materials for their antimicrobial properties, pose concerns regarding cytotoxicity and immunoreactivity. In a key study, Niska et al. (2016) used gingival fibroblast-derived organoids to investigate the effects of AgNPs with distinct surface modifications. The results demonstrated that nanoparticle capping agents markedly influenced both antimicrobial potency and cytotoxic potential, emphasizing the importance of assessing material biocompatibility within complex tissue-like models. Organoid-based testing thus provides a critical means to balance microbial control with host tissue safety in dental biomaterial development. Beyond biomaterials, organoids have emerged as powerful tools for preclinical evaluation of dental therapeutics, including antibiotics, anti-inflammatory agents, local anesthetics, and remineralization treatments. Traditional drug testing platforms often fail to mimic barrier properties, metabolic activity, and cellular interplay within oral tissues, leading to inconsistent or suboptimal therapeutic performance. Organoids derived from oral mucosa, gingiva, and dental pulp allow detailed analysis of drug penetration, retention, and cytotoxicity. Fluoride-containing remineralization agents, for example, have been tested in enamel–pulp organoid systems to examine their ability to traverse dentinal tubules and induce mineral deposition without compromising pulp cell viability. Similarly, antibiotics used in periodontal therapy have been evaluated in organoid-biofilm co-culture systems, enabling the study of antimicrobial efficacy, biofilm resistance, and interactions with host cells.

Advances in organoid research have also accelerated the development of sophisticated drug delivery systems. Nanoparticle-based carriers, liposomal formulations, and hydrogel-encapsulated therapeutics can be tested directly within dental pulp or oral mucosal organoids to model targeted release, uptake dynamics, and therapeutic efficacy. Organoid studies have demonstrated sustained release profiles, enhanced antibacterial activity, and reduced cytotoxicity for encapsulated drug formulations, validating their potential before *in vivo* application.

Despite these notable advances, several challenges remain in the integration of organoid systems into mainstream dental research. A persistent limitation is the lack of intrinsic vascularization, which constrains organoid size, metabolic complexity, and long-term viability. These factors are crucial for accurate drug metabolism and toxicity studies. To address this, microfluidic "organ-on-chip" systems are increasingly being incorporated to simulate perfusion, nutrient exchange, and waste removal, thereby enhancing physiological relevance. Additionally, variability in culture conditions across laboratories underscores the need for standardized protocols to improve reproducibility, scalability, and suitability for high-throughput drug screening.

2.13 SUMMARY

This chapter delineates how 3D organoid technology is advancing regenerative endodontics by providing models that closely reproduce the structural organization and multicellular interactions of dental tissues. Organoids derived from DPSCs, SHED, and SCAP demonstrate strong regenerative and odontogenic potential, enabling controlled investigations of pulp–dentin biology. The integration of biomimetic scaffolds, such as hydrogels and bioactive glass composites, together with signaling molecules like TGF-β1, enhances cellular differentiation, matrix remodeling, and tissue-specific functionality. The application of emerging fabrication approaches, including 3D bioprinting and microfluidic encapsulation, has further enabled the construction of vascularized and anatomically relevant organoid systems. These platforms are increasingly used to model pulpal and periapical inflammation, immune–stromal dynamics, and reparative processes and provide robust tools for evaluating biomaterials and therapeutic agents. Collectively, this chapter presents 3D organoids as a pivotal technological advance with substantial implications for the future of dental tissue engineering and regenerative endodontic therapy.

REFERENCES

Ayoub, C. G., Aminoshariae, A., Bakkar, M., Ghosh, S., Bonfield, T., Demko, C., Montagnese, T. A., & Mickel, A. K. (2017). Comparison of IL-1β, TNF-α, hBD-2, and hBD-3 expression in the dental pulp of smokers versus nonsmokers. *Journal of Endodontics*, 43(12), 2009–2013.

Chang, H. H., Chen, I. L., Wang, Y. L., Chang, M. C., Tsai, Y. L., Lan, W. C., & Wang, T. M. (2020). TGF-β1 regulates regenerative activity of dental pulp stem cells from exfoliated deciduous teeth through ALK5/Smad2, TAK1, p38, and MEK/ERK signaling pathways. *Stem Cells International*, 2020, 1565912.

Duka, M., Eraković, M., Dolićanin, Z., Stefanović, D., & Čolić, M. (2019, Mar 18). Production of soluble receptor activator of nuclear factor kappa-B ligand and osteoprotegerin by apical periodontitis cells in culture and their modulation by cytokines. *Mediators of Inflammation*, 2019, 8325380. doi: 10.1155/2019/8325380.

Duval, K., Grover, H., Han, L. H., Mou, Y., Pegoraro, A. F., Fredberg, J., & Chen, Z. (2017). Modeling physiological events in 2D vs. 3D cell culture. *Physiology*, 32(4), 266–277.

Edmondson, R., Broglie, J. J., Adcock, A. F., & Yang, L. (2014). Three-dimensional cell culture systems and their applications in drug discovery and cell-based biosensors. *ASSAY and Drug Development Technologies*, 12(4), 207–218.

Han, Y., Xu, J., Chopra, H., Zhang, Z., Dubey, N., Dissanayaka, W. L., Nör, J. E., & Bottino, M. C. (2024). Injectable tissue-specific hydrogel system for pulp-dentin regeneration. *Journal of Dental Research*, 103(4), 398–408.

Huang, G. T. J., Yamaza, T., & Shea, L. D. (2010). Stem/progenitor cell-mediated de novo regeneration of dental pulp with newly deposited dentin in an in vivo model. *Tissue Engineering Part A*, 16(7), 2063–2071.

Huang, Y., Tang, Y., Zhang, R. et al. (2024). Role of periodontal ligament fibroblasts in periodontitis: pathological mechanisms and therapeutic potential. *Journal of Translational Medicine*, 22, 1136. https://doi.org/10.1186/s12967-024-05944-8.

Kim, J. Y., Xin, X., Moioli, E. K., Chung, J., Lee, C. H., & Chen, M. (2021). Dental pulp organoids for regenerative endodontics. *Biomolecules*, 13(6), 1123.

Krivanek, J., Buchtova, M., Fried, K., & Adameyko, I. (2023). Plasticity of dental cell types in development, regeneration, and evolution. *Journal of Dental Research*, 102(6), 589–598.

Li, F. C., & Kishen, A. (2023). Development of dental pulp organoids for regenerative endodontics. *Biomolecules*, 13(6), 900.

Niska, K., Knap, N., Kędzia, A., Jaskiewicz, M., Kamysz, W., & Inkielewicz-Stepniak, I. (2016). Capping agent-dependent toxicity and antimicrobial activity of silver nanoparticles: An in vitro study. *International Journal of Medical Sciences*, 13(10), 772–782.

Sadaghiani, L., Mahmoudian, M., Sadighi, M., & Nekoofar, M. H. (2016). Conditioning of dental pulp stem cells: Effects of parathyroid hormone and vitamin D on differentiation and mineralization. *International Endodontic Journal*, 49(4), 376–387.

Tibbitt, M. W., & Anseth, K. S. (2009). Hydrogels as extracellular matrix mimics for 3D cell culture. *Biotechnology and Bioengineering*, 103(4), 655–663.

Wu, J., Mao, S., Xu, L., Qiu, D., Wang, S., & Dong, Y. (2022). Odontogenic differentiation induced by TGF-β1 binding peptide-modified bioglass. *Journal of Dental Research*, 101(10), 1190–1197.

Yamamoto, K., Sugita, Y., Kamata, Y., & Umezawa, K. (2020). Spheroid culture enhances the odontogenic differentiation capacity of human dental pulp stem cells. *Journal of Biomedical Materials Research Part A*, 108(7), 1676–1685.

Zhang, W., Jin, H., Lou, S., Yang, H., Dai, X., & Ma, S. (2024). Microfluidic droplet encapsulation-guided organoid growth promotes parental tumor phenotype recapitulation. *International Journal of Cancer*, 154(1), 145–154.

Zhang, W., Li, J., Zhou, J., Rastogi, A., & Ma, S. (2022). Translational organoid technology – The convergence of chemical, mechanical, and computational biology. *Trends in Biotechnology*, 40(9), 1121–1135.

Zhang, X., Zhang, S., Chen, H., & Ma, L. (2024). Advances in microfluidic systems for organoid culture: Applications in cancer research and tissue engineering. *Frontiers in Bioengineering and Biotechnology*, 12, 1356580.

Zhao, F., Zhang, Z., & Guo, W. (2024). The 3D printing for dental tissue regeneration: The state of the art and future challenges. *Frontiers in Bioengineering and Biotechnology*, 12, 1356580.

Chapter 3

Advances in 3D bioprinting for dental applications

3.1 INTRODUCTION

Despite significant advancements in biomaterials, diagnostic imaging, and clinical workflows, contemporary dentistry continues to face substantial biological and procedural challenges that limit predictable and minimally invasive patient care. Many restorative and regenerative interventions still rely on techniques that require extensive modifications of dental hard and soft tissues. These challenges span endodontics, periodontics, implantology, and oral rehabilitation, emphasizing the need for technologies capable of delivering precise tissue reconstruction with reduced iatrogenic damage. A large proportion of conventional dental procedures remain inherently invasive. Endodontic treatment, periodontal surgeries, and implant placement require surgical access and mechanical instrumentation that can compromise surrounding tissues. In implant dentistry, inadequate alveolar bone frequently necessitates adjunctive procedures such as ridge augmentation or sinus floor elevation, adding both complexity and biological burden to the treatment pathway. These interventions increase the risk of postoperative inflammation, infection, graft failure, and impaired osseointegration, while also prolonging healing times and contributing to patient morbidity (Turkyilmaz and Wilkins, 2021). The need to reduce surgical trauma without compromising functional outcomes remains a central clinical priority.

This context underscores the importance of developing therapeutic strategies that are both biologically informed and minimally invasive. Approaches that enable precise spatial control over tissue reconstruction, preserve native structures, and support physiological healing responses are of particular relevance. Three-dimensional (3D) bioprinting represents a promising technological platform in this regard, offering the ability to fabricate anatomically accurate, biomimetic constructs that can be customized to patient-specific geometries. By integrating advanced biomaterials, engineered bioinks, and computational design frameworks, bioprinting provides a pathway toward regenerative solutions that may overcome the limitations of conventional dental procedures and advance the clinical management of oral and craniofacial tissues.

DOI: 10.1201/9781003589921-3

The biomaterials currently used in dental practice, although effective within defined clinical parameters, exhibit intrinsic limitations that restrict their long-term performance. Amalgam restorations demonstrate considerable durability but remain under scrutiny due to their mercury content and the associated environmental and toxicological concerns. Ceramic-based materials provide excellent esthetics and biocompatibility; however, their intrinsic brittleness renders them susceptible to catastrophic fracture under high occlusal loads. Composite resins offer greater versatility and improved handling, yet their polymer-based matrices frequently exhibit inadequate mechanical strength and susceptibility to wear, jeopardizing the longevity of restorations (Dawood et al., 2015). Furthermore, conventionally used biomaterials seldom exhibit true biological integration with host tissues. The absence of biomimetic properties contributes to complications such as microleakage at restoration margins, limited osseointegration in implant dentistry, and the progressive mechanical failure of prosthetic rehabilitations. These deficits highlight the critical need for next-generation materials capable of replicating the hierarchical structure, mechanical resilience, and biological responsiveness of native dental tissues.

Periodontal diseases, which compromise gingiva and supporting connective and osseous structures, remain one of the most prevalent causes of tooth loss globally. Current therapeutic strategies primarily focus on reducing inflammation and controlling microbial infection, but they provide limited capacity for regenerating the complex architecture of lost periodontal tissues. Likewise, the restoration of alveolar bone in cases of advanced resorption continues to pose significant clinical difficulty. Traditional grafting procedures, despite their widespread use, require extensive surgical manipulation and carry risks including donor site morbidity, graft rejection, and unpredictable healing dynamics (Rasperini et al., 2015). The development of regenerative technologies that support endogenous tissue repair, such as bioactive scaffolds, advanced hydrogel systems, and controlled growth factor delivery platforms, has therefore become a central focus in periodontal and bone regeneration research. 3D bioprinting holds promise by enabling the fabrication of custom-engineered scaffolds with precise microarchitectures that facilitate cellular infiltration, vascularization, and functional tissue regeneration.

Recovery periods associated with many dental interventions remain another significant clinical barrier. Surgical procedures such as extractions, implant placement, and bone augmentation are often followed by prolonged healing phases, delaying the restoration of masticatory function and negatively influencing patient well-being. Slow tissue regeneration increases susceptibility to postoperative complications, including infection, graft resorption, and early implant instability. Accelerating the healing cascade while maintaining structural and functional outcomes is therefore a critical objective in contemporary dental research. Bioprinting technologies, which allow the incorporation of progenitor cells, biomimetic matrices, and bioactive signaling molecules into 3D constructs, offer a viable means of promoting rapid tissue regeneration. These engineered systems have the potential to reduce healing times substantially and improve clinical predictability by fostering early cell recruitment, enhanced matrix deposition, and accelerated functional integration of engineered tissues.

3.2 THREE-DIMENSIONAL BIOPRINTING AND ITS EMERGING ROLE IN DENTAL THERAPEUTICS

Within dentistry, the 3D bioprinting provides an unprecedented capability to fabricate complex, patient-specific constructs that overcome the inherent limitations of conventional restorative and regenerative techniques. By enabling the spatially controlled deposition of living cells, biomimetic biomaterials, and bioactive signaling molecules, bioprinting supports the generation of functional tissues, engineered scaffolds, and prosthetic components tailored to individual clinical needs.

Unlike conventional 3D printing, which relies on polymers, metals, or ceramics for structural fabrication, 3D bioprinting employs bioinks composed of viable cells, extracellular matrix (ECM)-mimicking hydrogels, growth factors, and composite biomaterials. These bioinks are extruded or polymerized layer by layer to form 3D constructs that closely resemble the architecture and biological properties of native dental and craniofacial tissues. This capacity to produce biologically active structures positions bioprinting as an important tool for advancing dental regeneration, enhancing implant integration, and enabling the development of next-generation tissue models for research and therapeutic applications.

3.2.1 Fundamentals of three-dimensional bioprinting

3D bioprinting provides a platform for the precise fabrication of biologically functional constructs capable of addressing complex oral and craniofacial challenges (Table 3.1). By integrating principles of additive manufacturing with cell-laden bioengineering strategies, this technology enables the construction of dental tissues and scaffolds with superior spatial fidelity and biological relevance. A range of bioprinting modalities have emerged, each offering distinct operational mechanisms and advantages for specific dental applications. Understanding the fundamental approaches, inkjet bioprinting, stereolithography, digital light processing, and fused deposition modeling is essential for selecting and optimizing the appropriate technology for regenerative and restorative interventions. Collectively, these modalities illustrate how 3D bioprinting can be tailored to fabricate constructs suited to diverse clinical and research objectives within dentistry (Figure 3.1).

Table 3.1 Comparison of 3D bioprinting techniques for dental applications

Bioprinting technique	*Mechanism*	*Advantages*	*Limitations*	*Applications in dentistry*
Inkjet bioprinting	Thermal or piezoelectric actuators deposit droplets of bioink	High resolution, suitable for soft tissues	Limited to low-viscosity bioinks	Periodontal tissue scaffolds and pulp regeneration
Stereolithography (SLA)	UV laser cures photosensitive resins layer by layer	High precision and smooth surface finish	Limited to photopolymer-based materials	Dental crowns, bridges, and surgical guides
Digital light processing (DLP)	Projected light cures entire layers simultaneously	Faster than SLA and maintains high resolution	Material selection limited to resins	Orthodontic aligners and custom trays
Fused deposition modeling (FDM)	Thermoplastic filaments extruded layer by layer	Cost-effective and mechanically strong	High temperatures limit bioink use	Mold fabrication and dental frameworks
Extrusion-based bioprinting	Pneumatic or mechanical extrusion of bioinks	Supports cell-laden bioinks	Lower resolution than SLA/DLP	3D tissue constructs and scaffolds for bone regeneration

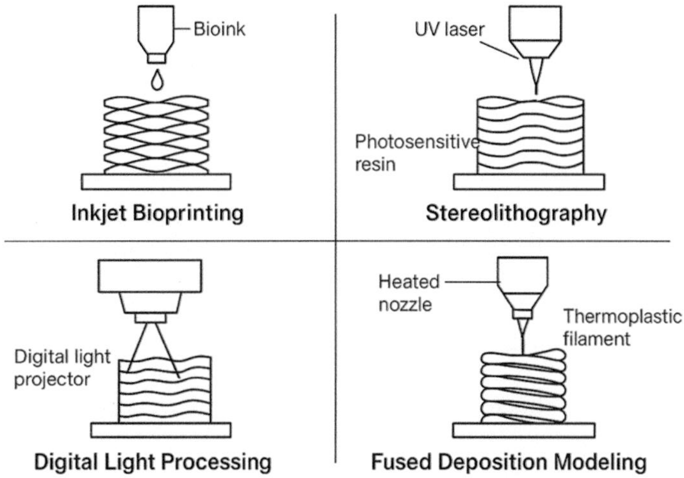

Figure 3.1 Major bioprinting modalities used in dental tissue engineering. A comparative overview illustrating the mechanisms, advantages, and dental applications of inkjet bioprinting, SLA, DLP, and FDM.

3.2.1.1 Inkjet bioprinting

Inkjet bioprinting employs thermal or piezoelectric actuation to dispense discrete droplets of bioink onto a substrate in precisely controlled patterns. This noncontact, high-resolution technique is particularly advantageous for depositing growth factors, low-viscosity hydrogels, and cell suspensions with minimal shear stress on embedded cells (Murphy and Atala, 2014). In dentistry, inkjet systems have been explored for fabricating scaffolds for periodontal regeneration, where growth factor-enriched hydrogels can support coordinated soft and hard tissue healing (Rasperini et al., 2015). Despite its precision, the requirement for low-viscosity bioinks limits the range of biomaterials that can be employed, constraining the mechanical robustness of printed constructs. This limitation prompts the use of complementary bioprinting modalities capable of processing more viscous or structurally stable biomaterials.

3.2.1.2 Stereolithography (SLA)

Stereolithography utilizes a focused ultraviolet laser to polymerize photosensitive resins in a layer-by-layer manner, producing structures with exceptional accuracy and surface smoothness. SLA has been widely adopted in dentistry for fabricating crowns, bridges, surgical guides, and high-fidelity anatomical models (Dawood et al., 2015). Its ability to generate intricate geometries with minimal post-processing makes SLA particularly suitable for precision-dependent applications such as implant planning and prosthodontic reconstruction. However, because SLA relies primarily on photopolymerizable resins, its direct application to cell-laden bioprinting remains limited, necessitating alternative light-based approaches for biological constructs.

3.2.1.3 Digital light processing (DLP)

DLP builds upon the principles of SLA by using a projected light pattern to cure entire resin layers simultaneously. This parallel curing mechanism significantly accelerates fabrication speed while maintaining high resolution (Chen et al., 2020). Within dentistry, DLP is especially valuable for producing orthodontic aligners, custom trays, occlusal devices, and rapid chairside prototypes. The method's efficiency and geometric precision make it particularly advantageous in orthodontics, where timely fabrication and accurate reproduction of dental morphology are essential. As light-based bioprinting technologies advance, DLP-adapted systems are being investigated for bioink curing, creating opportunities for future applications in regenerative tissue constructs.

3.2.1.4 *Fused deposition modeling (FDM)*

FDM constructs 3D structures by extruding thermoplastic filaments through a heated nozzle in a controlled, layer-wise fashion. Although traditional FDM operates at temperatures incompatible with living cells and is therefore less suitable for direct bioprinting, it remains widely used in dentistry for producing robust molds, splints, frameworks, and educational prototypes (Ventola, 2014). Recent research has focused on adapting FDM platforms to process composite biomaterials and temperature-responsive polymers, enabling the fabrication of scaffolds with enhanced mechanical strength for bone and periodontal regeneration. These developments position FDM as a complementary technique that can support hybrid bioprinting workflows.

3.2.2 Materials used in three-dimensional bioprinting for dental applications

The choice of materials for 3D bioprinting is pivotal to achieving functional, clinically relevant constructs in dental and craniofacial regeneration (Table 3.2). These materials, collectively referred to as bioinks and structural components, must exhibit a combination of biological compatibility, tunable mechanical strength, and reliable printability. In dental applications, where tissues range from soft (pulp and gingiva) to highly mineralized (dentin and bone), material selection becomes especially critical. The principal classes of materials used include hydrogels, ceramics, and composite formulations, each offering unique advantages that can be strategically combined to meet complex biological and mechanical requirements (Figure 3.2).

3.2.2.1 *Hydrogels*

Hydrogels constitute the foundational class of bioinks due to their high water content, biocompatibility, and ability to mimic the ECM. Their hydrated polymer networks support cell encapsulation, nutrient exchange, and tissue-specific differentiation, making them indispensable for soft-tissue applications in dental bioprinting.

A. Alginate: Alginate, derived from brown seaweed, is widely utilized for its rapid ionic crosslinking and mild gelation properties. When crosslinked with divalent cations such as calcium, alginate forms structurally stable hydrogels suitable for bioprinting. It has been extensively applied in dental pulp regeneration and periodontal scaffolding owing to its cytocompatibility and ease of processing (Ong et al., 2017).
B. Gelatin: Gelatin-based hydrogels provide natural cell adhesion motifs that promote cell attachment and proliferation. Their methacrylated

Table 3.2 Bioinks used in 3D bioprinting for dental applications

Bioink type	*Composition*	*Key properties*	*Applications in dentistry*
Hydrogels	Alginate, gelatin, and chitosan	High biocompatibility; supports cell encapsulation	Pulp–dentin regeneration and periodontal scaffolds
Ceramics	Hydroxyapatite (HA) and tricalcium phosphate (TCP)	Promotes osseointegration and mimics bone	Alveolar bone regeneration and dental implants
Composites	Hydrogel-ceramic mixtures and polymer blends	Combines flexibility with mechanical strength	Multitissue scaffolds and periodontal regeneration
Nanocomposites	Nanoparticles (e.g., carbon nanotubes and silica)	Enhances mechanical properties and antimicrobial effects	Dental restorations and bioactive coatings
Hybrid bioinks	Combination of synthetic and natural polymers	Improved cell adhesion and tailored degradation rates	Multimaterial scaffolds for complex tissue engineering

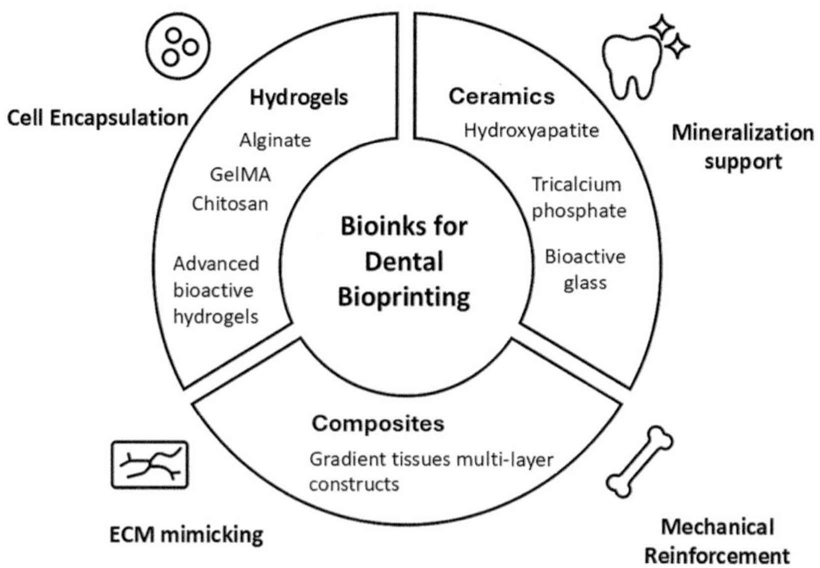

Figure 3.2 Bioinks applied in dental bioprinting and their functional roles. The diagram categorizes hydrogels, ceramics, and composite systems used in dental regeneration. It illustrates their mechanical properties, biological functions, and tissue-specific relevance, including applications in pulp, periodontal ligament, dentin, and alveolar bone engineering.

derivatives, particularly gelatin methacrylate (GelMA), offer enhanced mechanical strength and controlled photopolymerization, enabling the printing of constructs requiring structural coherence (Chen et al., 2020).

C. Chitosan: Chitosan, a chitin-derived biopolymer, is valued for its antimicrobial properties and biodegradability. Its incorporation into hydrogel systems enhances scaffold bioactivity and has shown significant potential in periodontal and alveolar bone regeneration (Murphy and Atala, 2014).

D. Advanced Hydrogels: Recent advancements integrate nanoparticles, growth factors, and signaling peptides into hydrogel matrices, resulting in bioinks with improved mechanical resilience, biological responsiveness, and controlled therapeutic release. These next-generation hydrogels are increasingly applied in complex dental tissue engineering and drug delivery strategies (Rasperini et al., 2015).

Together, hydrogel systems form the biological basis of many dental bioprinting strategies, but their limited mechanical strength often necessitates reinforcement through ceramic or polymeric components.

3.2.2.2 Ceramics

Ceramic materials play an important role in bioprinting constructs intended for hard-tissue regeneration. Their bioactive behavior, mineral composition, and similarity to the inorganic matrix of bone and dental tissues make them invaluable for applications involving alveolar bone, cementum, and dentin repair.

A. Hydroxyapatite (HA): HA, the principal mineral component of bone and teeth, is widely incorporated into dental scaffolds to promote osteoconduction and osseointegration. Its biological affinity for natural tissues makes it one of the most extensively studied ceramics for alveolar bone regeneration (Murphy and Atala, 2020).

B. Tricalcium Phosphate (TCP): TCP exhibits controlled biodegradability and supports the physiological processes of bone remodeling. When combined with hydrogels or polymeric materials, TCP enhances scaffold mechanical properties and biological performance (Ong et al., 2017).

C. Bioactive Glass: Bioactive glass possesses exceptional regenerative capacity, forming strong bonds with hard and soft tissues. Its ionic dissolution products stimulate cellular activity and mineralization, making it a promising candidate for periodontal, alveolar bone, and even enamel regeneration (Rasperini et al., 2015).

Ceramics therefore provide the structural stiffness and mineral cues necessary for engineering load-bearing constructs, complementing the biological functions of hydrogels.

3.2.2.3 *Composites*

Composite bioinks integrate the benefits of hydrogels, ceramics, and polymers to produce multifunctional materials capable of supporting both biological activity and mechanical demands. These hybrid systems are particularly suited for dental bioprinting applications involving gradient tissues or a multilayered architectures.

A. Hydrogel–Ceramic Composites: Blending hydrogels with ceramic particles such as HA or TCP enhances mechanical stability while preserving cell-friendly environments. These composites are ideal for alveolar bone and periodontal regeneration, where both biological integration and load-bearing capacity are required (Chen et al., 2020).
B. Nanocomposites: The incorporation of nanomaterials, including carbon nanotubes, silica nanoparticles, and nano-hydroxyapatite, into bioinks significantly improves mechanical performance, electrical conductivity, and biological signaling. Nanocomposite bioinks are being actively explored for dental restorative materials and implant coatings (Murphy and Atala, 2014).
C. Hybrid Systems: Hybrid composites integrating hydrogels, ceramics, and biodegradable polymers offer the highest versatility. Their tunable porosity, mechanical strength, and biological functionality enable their use in multifaceted dental applications, such as simultaneous regeneration of alveolar bone, periodontal ligament, and cementum (Ong et al., 2017).

Collectively, composite materials bridge the gap between soft- and hard-tissue engineering, enabling the fabrication of anatomically and functionally integrated dental constructs.

3.2.3 Scaffolds and structural materials

Scaffolds and structural materials constitute the architectural backbone of 3D bioprinting strategies for dental applications. Their primary function is to provide mechanical stability, spatial guidance, and a biologically conducive microenvironment to support cell adhesion, proliferation, and tissue maturation. The choice of scaffold materials profoundly influences tissue regeneration outcomes by dictating mechanical strength, degradation kinetics, biocompatibility, and integration with native oral tissues. Within dental tissue engineering, key classes of scaffold materials include synthetic biodegradable polymers, natural polymers, and composite formulations optimized for hard- and soft-tissue regeneration.

3.2.3.1 *Polycaprolactone (PCL)*

PCL is a semicrystalline, biodegradable polyester widely adopted in dental and craniofacial tissue engineering due to its advantageous mechanical properties, ease of fabrication, and predictable long-term degradation profile. PCL scaffolds can be produced using extrusion-based 3D printing, enabling precise control over pore geometry, interconnectivity, and mechanical behavior. Recent innovations have centered on improving PCL's inherently limited bioactivity. Moghaddaszadeh et al. (2021) demonstrated that integrating carbonated nanohydroxyapatite and immobilized collagen into a 3D-printed PCL framework significantly enhanced its physicomechanical properties and osteoconductive potential. Such biomimetic reinforcement positions PCL-based scaffolds as promising candidates for alveolar bone regeneration and load-bearing dental applications.

3.2.3.2 Polylactic-co-glycolic acid (PLGA)

PLGA is a copolymer known for its biodegradability and biocompatibility, making it suitable for various biomedical applications, including dental scaffolds. Its degradation rate can be tailored by adjusting the ratio of lactic to glycolic acid, allowing for controlled resorption that matches tissue healing rates. Ge et al. (2009) investigated the proliferation and differentiation of human osteoblasts within 3D-printed PLGA scaffolds, demonstrating that these scaffolds possess mechanical properties similar to those of trabecular bone and support osteoblast activity, indicating their potential for bone regeneration in dental applications.

3.2.3.3 Collagen-based scaffolds

Collagen, being a major component of the ECM, offers excellent biocompatibility and promotes cell adhesion and proliferation. In dental tissue engineering, collagen-based scaffolds are often used to mimic the natural tissue environment. Han et al. (2024) developed an injectable tissue-specific hydrogel system using collagen for pulp–dentin regeneration. Their study demonstrated that dental pulp stem cells encapsulated in a collagen-based hydrogel with varying stiffness could regenerate functional dental pulp and dentin when injected into tooth slices, highlighting the potential of collagen-based scaffolds in regenerative endodontics.

3.2.3.4 Composite scaffolds

Combining different materials to form composite scaffolds can leverage the advantages of each component, resulting in enhanced mechanical strength and bioactivity. For example, incorporating HA or other bioactive ceramics into polymer matrices like PCL or PLGA can improve osteo-conductivity and mechanical properties. Such composite scaffolds are particularly useful in dental applications requiring the regeneration of hard tissues like bone. The integration of bioactive nanoparticles into polymeric scaffolds has also been explored to further enhance their functionality.

3.3 SURFACE MODIFICATION TECHNIQUES

Modifying the surface characteristics of scaffolds is a critical strategy for improving cellular responses and promoting successful tissue integration. Surface engineering approaches such as immobilization of bioactive molecules, plasma treatment, and coating with ECM components have been widely employed to enhance cell adhesion, proliferation, and differentiation. For example, collagen-functionalized PCL scaffolds have been shown to significantly enhance osteoblast activity, improving early cell attachment and accelerating integration with adjacent bone tissue. Similarly, the incorporation of growth factors onto scaffold surfaces can direct lineage-specific differentiation, supporting more predictable outcomes in dental tissue engineering. Collectively, these surface modification strategies help bridge the gap between scaffold design and biological performance, improving the translational potential of bioprinted constructs (Figure 3.3).

3.3.1 Technical considerations in dental bioprinting

The successful clinical translation of 3D bioprinting for dental applications relies on overcoming several key technical challenges. These

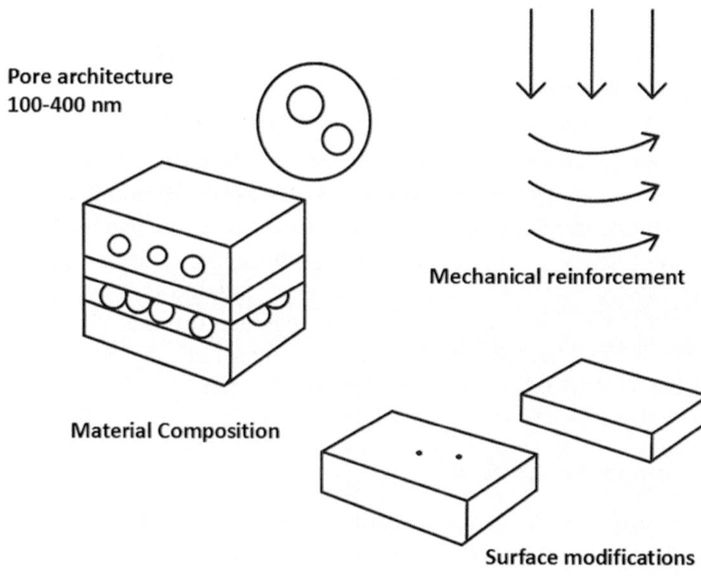

Figure 3.3 Essential scaffold design parameters for dental and periodontal tissue regeneration. This figure depicts architectural, mechanical, and biological design considerations for scaffolds, including pore geometry, gradient structures, load-bearing reinforcement, and surface functionalization that support hard- and soft-tissue regeneration.

considerations directly influence the accuracy, biocompatibility, and mechanical performance of bioprinted tissues and prosthetic structures, ultimately determining their feasibility for clinical use.

3.3.1.1 Resolution and precision

Dental tissues possess intricate microanatomy, including fine enamel prisms, periodontal ligament fibers, dentinal tubules, and complex pulp structures. Replicating these features requires high-resolution bioprinting technologies capable of producing micrometer-scale precision. SLA and DLP systems are widely used in dentistry because they can achieve layer resolutions approaching 25 microns (Chen et al., 2020). Such precision is essential for producing crowns, aligners, occlusal appliances, and detailed anatomical models that must conform to the 3D geometry of the oral cavity. Inaccuracies in printed constructs can lead to prosthetic misfits, discomfort, biological complications, or failure of regenerative scaffolds. High-resolution fabrication has been shown to improve scaffold performance in periodontal and alveolar bone tissue engineering by enhancing tissue-scaffold integration and reducing the risk of mechanical or structural failure (Rasperini et al., 2015).

3.3.2 Biocompatibility

Biocompatibility remains a primary requirement for all bioprinted dental materials. Bioinks must avoid eliciting inflammatory reactions, immune rejection, or cytotoxicity. Compliance with regulatory frameworks established by agencies such as the Food and Drug Administration and European Medicines Agency is essential. Standard bioinks, including hydrogels, composites, and natural polymers, undergo extensive biological testing to ensure safety and efficacy (Murphy and Atala, 2014). During bioprinting, cells may be exposed to shear forces, temperature fluctuations, and mechanical stress that can compromise viability. Advances in bioink design, such as shear-thinning hydrogels, thermosensitive matrices, and viscoelastic polymer blends, have significantly improved the preservation of cell function throughout the printing process (Ong et al., 2017). Maintaining sterility during printing is equally critical. Bioprinters used in regenerative dentistry typically operate in controlled sterile environments, with all consumables sterilized via gamma irradiation, autoclaving, or low-temperature methods to prevent microbial contamination (Rasperini et al., 2015).

3.3.3 Mechanical properties

Dental tissues are routinely exposed to substantial mechanical loads generated during mastication, speech, and parafunctional activity. Human enamel exhibits a compressive strength of approximately 384 MPa, whereas the periodontal ligament demonstrates a tensile strength near 4 MPa

(Ong et al., 2017). To achieve long-term functional stability, bioprinted scaffolds and implantable prosthetics must approximate these native mechanical properties. Importantly, the mechanical requirements vary across dental tissues, scaffolds for alveolar bone regeneration must possess high compressive stiffness to withstand occlusal forces, while those intended for gingival or periodontal ligament repair require greater elasticity to support physiological soft-tissue motion. Composite scaffolds incorporating polymers such as PCL with mineral phases like HA are frequently employed to achieve this balance, providing both structural resilience and enhanced osteoconductivity (Chen et al., 2020). In addition to mechanical loading, scaffolds must remain stable in the dynamic and chemically variable conditions of the oral cavity, which is characterized by pH fluctuations, enzymatic activity, microbial biofilms, and continuous mechanical abrasion. Biodegradable polymers such as PCL and PLA are widely used due to their predictable degradation profiles and resistance to hydrolytic breakdown, enabling gradual scaffold resorption while maintaining sufficient structural integrity during tissue maturation (Murphy and Atala, 2020).

3.3.4 Printability

The rheological properties of bioinks are central to determining their printability, extrusion behavior, and post-deposition stability. Ideal bioinks exhibit shear-thinning behavior, enabling smooth flow through the nozzle under applied shear stress and rapid viscosity recovery upon deposition to maintain structural fidelity. Bioinks with excessively high viscosity can obstruct nozzle flow and compromise cell viability, while those with very low viscosity may diffuse uncontrollably, leading to poor layer definition and loss of architectural precision (Murphy and Atala, 2014). Post-printing stabilization relies on effective crosslinking mechanisms that reinforce the construct's mechanical and biological performance. Common strategies include photopolymerization using ultraviolet (UV) light, ionic crosslinking such as calcium-mediated gelation of alginates, and thermally induced gelation for temperature-responsive bioinks, each providing tunable control over scaffold stiffness and integrity (Chen et al., 2020). Multimaterial bioprinting further expands the capabilities of dental tissue engineering by enabling the coordinated deposition of diverse bioinks within a single construct. This approach allows the fabrication of heterogeneous architectures that more closely mimic the compositional and mechanical gradients of natural dental tissues. For instance, rigid, mineral-rich bioinks can be used to reproduce dentin or alveolar bone regions, while softer hydrogels may be simultaneously printed to regenerate pulp or periodontal ligament tissues, supporting integrated multitissue regeneration within a unified scaffold (Rasperini et al., 2015).

3.3.5 Post-processing and functionalization

Post-processing strategies play a critical role in enhancing the biological performance of bioprinted constructs. Surface functionalization techniques, such as coating scaffolds with ECM components or immobilizing growth factors, can significantly improve cell adhesion, proliferation, and lineage-specific differentiation. Collagen-functionalized scaffolds, for instance, have been shown to enhance osteoblast activity and promote more effective integration with host bone tissue (Ong et al., 2017). In addition to biological augmentation, post-processing must also ensure sterility without compromising scaffold structure or bioactivity. Sterilization methods such as ethylene oxide treatment and gamma irradiation are commonly employed; however, these approaches must be carefully optimized to avoid adverse effects on polymer integrity or denaturation of incorporated bioactive molecules (Murphy and Atala, 2014).

3.4 APPLICATIONS OF THREE-DIMENSIONAL BIOPRINTING IN DENTISTRY

The use of 3D bioprinting in dentistry spans a wide range of clinical and research applications, including prosthetic design, periodontal regeneration, tissue-engineered implant interfaces, and orthodontic innovations (Table 3.3). By integrating patient-specific imaging, computer-aided design, and advanced biomaterials, bioprinting offers unprecedented precision and customization in the fabrication of dental structures.

Table 3.3 Applications of 3D bioprinting in dentistry

Applications	*Description*	*Example*
Dental prosthetics	Fabrication of crowns, bridges, and dentures with enhanced precision	SLA-printed dental crowns with custom fit
Periodontal regeneration	Bioengineered scaffolds for gum tissue repair	3D-printed hydrogel scaffolds for periodontitis treatment
Tissue engineering for implants	Bioactive scaffolds for improved osseointegration	PCL–HA composite implants for alveolar bone regeneration
Orthodontics	Custom fabrication of aligners and brackets	DLP-printed clear aligners for orthodontic treatment
Drug and biomaterial testing	*In vitro* models for evaluating the biocompatibility	3D-bioprinted pulp organoids for endodontic material testing

3.4.1 Fabrication of dental prosthetics

3D bioprinting has significantly transformed prosthetic fabrication by enabling rapid, precise, and anatomically accurate replication of dental structures. Conventional manufacturing of crowns, bridges, and dentures is often labor-intensive and susceptible to inaccuracies, especially during manual impression-taking and casting. In contrast, bioprinting integrated with digital workflows allows the automated fabrication of prosthetics with high fidelity and reduced turnaround times. SLA and DLP have emerged as dominant technologies for producing crowns and bridges using biocompatible photopolymer resins. These methods generate prosthetics with exceptionally smooth surface finishes, minimizing post-processing requirements and improving marginal adaptation (Chen et al., 2020). For complete dentures, bioprinting enables simultaneous fabrication of the denture base and teeth, resulting in superior fit, improved comfort, and reduced clinical chair time. Studies have demonstrated that bioprinted denture bases exhibit mechanical properties comparable to those produced using conventional acrylic resins, with the added advantage of enhanced customization (Murphy et al., 2014).

3.4.2 Customization and precision in prosthetic design

Personalized prosthetic design is a cornerstone of modern digital dentistry. Using computer-aided design (CAD) platforms, clinicians can tailor prosthetics to patient-specific anatomy derived from cone-beam computed tomography (CBCT) and intraoral scans. Bioprinting strengthens this workflow by enabling the precise reproduction of these digital designs with micrometer-scale accuracy. A significant advancement in this area is multimaterial bioprinting, which allows different materials to be deposited within a single prosthetic unit. This capability is particularly valuable for replicating the hierarchical structure of natural teeth, where an enamel-like material can be printed for the outer layer while a dentin-like resin provides supportive internal structure (Dawood et al., 2015). This biomimetic design approach enhances both the functional and esthetic outcomes of bioprinted prosthetics.

3.4.3 Development of periodontal scaffolds

Periodontal tissue engineering is one of the most promising applications of 3D bioprinting, given the multifactorial nature of periodontal diseases and the complexity of regenerating the gum–ligament–bone interface.

A. Regeneration of Gingival Soft Tissues: Periodontal diseases, such as chronic periodontitis, result in the destruction of gingival tissues and supporting alveolar bone. 3D bioprinting enables the fabrication of scaffolds that mimic the ECM, providing a biologically supportive environment for cell adhesion and differentiation. Hydrogels such as GelMA and alginate are frequently used due to their biocompatibility and tunable mechanical properties. Incorporation of growth factors such as platelet-derived growth factor further accelerates tissue regeneration. Rasperini et al. (2015) demonstrated that bioprinted scaffolds enhanced periodontal soft tissue repair, improving gingival thickness, connective tissue attachment, and overall periodontal stability.

B. Integration with Existing Dental Structures: Successful periodontal regeneration requires that the newly formed tissues integrate seamlessly with existing structures, including dental roots and remaining ligament fibers. To achieve this, bioprinted scaffolds can be engineered with gradient pore architectures that support vascularization and nutrient diffusion, which is essential for tissue survival (Ong et al., 2017). Additionally, surface modifications such as collagen coatings, ECM deposition, or bioactive peptide immobilization improve cellular attachment and facilitate strong integration between regenerated tissues and natural dental structures.

3.4.4 Tissue engineering for dental implants

3D bioprinting also plays a pivotal role in the advancement of next-generation dental implants by enabling biological integration and replacing traditional inert materials with biologically functional constructs.

A. Bioengineered Tooth Roots: The fabrication of bioengineered tooth roots represents a major step forward in implantology. Using bioprinting, scaffolds can be constructed with highly specific geometries that mimic natural root morphology, promoting appropriate cellular infiltration and mechanical function. Composite scaffolds incorporating PCL and HA provide both mechanical strength and biological cues essential for osteointegration (Chen et al., 2020). These biomimetic constructs offer the potential to replace titanium implants with biologically active alternatives capable of supporting natural tooth–bone interactions.

B. Osseointegration Challenges and Solutions: Achieving successful osseointegration remains a key challenge in implant dentistry, particularly in patients with compromised bone quality. 3D bioprinting addresses this challenge by enabling precise control over surface roughness, porosity, and microarchitecture. These parameters are known to influence osteoblast adhesion and bone ingrowth. Bioactive surface coatings incorporating osteogenic molecules, including bone morphogenetic proteins, have further improved osseointegration by stimulating early osteogenesis. Multimaterial bioprinting also allows the incorporation of bioactive ceramics such as tricalcium phosphate into implant frameworks, enhancing mineralization and long-term stability (Murphy and Atala, 2014).

3.4.5 Orthodontics

A. Fabrication of Aligners and Brackets: Orthodontics has been significantly advanced by the integration of 3D bioprinting technologies, particularly in the fabrication of clear aligners and customized brackets. Conventional aligner fabrication requires multiple manual steps, including vacuum forming, trimming, and polishing, which are prone to dimensional inaccuracies and extended chairside time. By contrast, 3D bioprinting enables direct fabrication from digital orthodontic models, streamlining production and improving precision. DLP is among the most widely deployed technologies for producing orthodontic aligners, owing to its ability to generate high-resolution constructs directly from CAD files. These aligners exhibit improved retention because they are tailored to each patient's dentition with micrometer-level accuracy (Dawood et al., 2015). Moreover, the rapid prototyping capacity of 3D bioprinting allows clinicians to generate successive aligners as the treatment progresses, enabling dynamic modifications without the delays associated with traditional laboratory workflows.

B. Improvements in Patient-Specific Orthodontic Devices: The customization advantages of 3D bioprinting extend beyond aligners to the design and fabrication of orthodontic brackets. Bioprinted brackets can be engineered to conform precisely to the anatomical contours of individual teeth, reducing the need for repositioning, minimizing bracket failure, and enhancing force transmission during tooth movement. Additionally, the ability to incorporate varied materials within a single design, which is not feasible with conventional bracket fabrication, allows for improved mechanical durability and patient comfort. Recent work has demonstrated that orthodontic brackets fabricated from biocompatible printed polymers exhibit high wear resistance, strong adhesive performance, and favorable biomechanical characteristics (Ong et al., 2017). The integration of CBCT data with bioprinting workflows further improves the precision and predictability of orthodontic appliances, ensuring more accurate bracket placement and optimized treatment outcomes (Figure 3.4).

3.5 ADVANCES IN 3D BIOPRINTING TECHNOLOGIES

3.5.1 Integration of AI and machine learning in 3D bioprinting workflows

Artificial intelligence (AI) and machine learning (ML) are increasingly reshaping 3D bioprinting, particularly within dental tissue engineering, by enabling more precise, adaptive, and scalable biomanufacturing

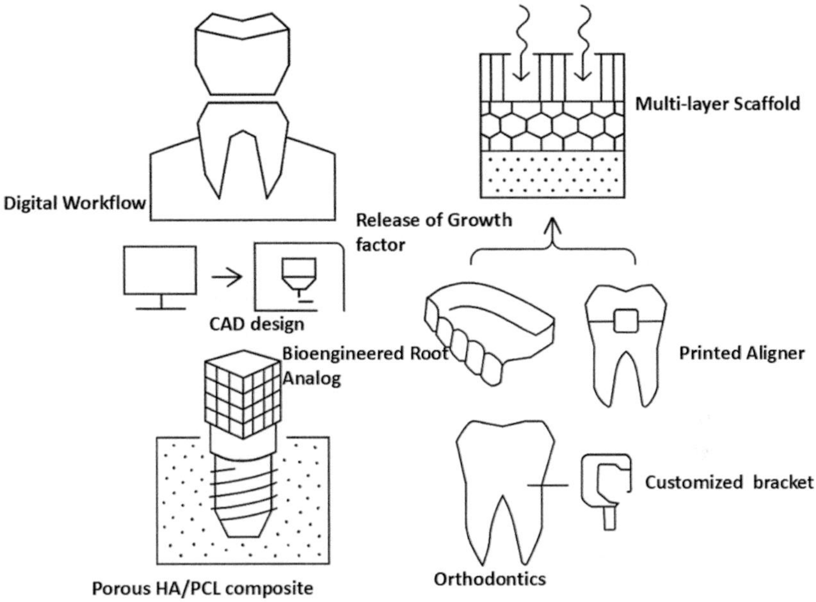

Figure 3.4 Clinical applications of 3D bioprinting across major dental specialties. A schematic illustrating how bioprinting supports prosthodontics, periodontal regeneration, implant engineering, and orthodontics. The figure highlights representative constructs such as prosthetic crowns, periodontal scaffolds, root analog implants, and patient-specific orthodontic devices.

workflows. AI-driven optimization algorithms can automatically refine critical printing parameters, such as extrusion pressure, nozzle temperature, print speed, and material flow rate, based on real-time input from sensors and historical datasets. These predictive models significantly reduce variability, improve construct fidelity, and enhance reproducibility across printing sessions (Nguyen et al., 2021). Beyond process optimization, AI facilitates the simulation of tissue growth and remodeling dynamics within bioprinted dental scaffolds. Such predictive frameworks allow researchers to visualize how engineered constructs will integrate with native tissues over time, enabling more precise design of patient-specific regenerative solutions. ML is also used to analyze micro-CT, optical coherence tomography, and CBCT imaging data from printed structures, providing automated feedback for iterative improvements in scaffold architecture (Santana et al., 2020). As bioprinting technologies evolve, the role of AI is expected to expand toward real-time error correction, autonomous quality control, and fully automated design-to-fabrication pipelines.

3.5.2 Innovations in bioink formulations for dental applications

The development of advanced bioinks is central to enabling functional, clinically relevant dental bioprinting. Modern bioinks often combine natural polymers such as alginate, gelatin, and collagen with synthetic materials including PEG, PCL derivatives, and polyurethane to achieve an optimal balance of printability, mechanical resilience, and biocompatibility. Hybrid bioinks have demonstrated superior adhesion, structural stability, and cell viability compared to single-component systems, making them well suited for regenerating enamel, dentin, pulp, and periodontal tissues (Wang et al., 2021). Nanotechnology has further expanded the utility of dental bioinks. Incorporation of nanoparticles, such as HA, silica, graphene oxide, and bioactive glass enhances mineralization, osteoconductivity, and mechanical strength, thereby improving the biomimetic qualities of printed dental constructs (Kim et al., 2020). Additionally, embedding signaling molecules such as growth factors, peptides, and morphogens into bioinks enables targeted differentiation of stem cells and accelerates tissue development. These innovations position next-generation bioinks as versatile platforms for sophisticated, multitissue dental regeneration.

3.5.3 High-resolution 3D bioprinters for complex dental structures

High-resolution bioprinting technologies are essential for replicating the fine anatomical features of dental and periodontal tissues. Advanced systems such as two-photon polymerization, micro-stereolithography, and refined DLP platforms can achieve sub-micron to micrometer-level precision, enabling fabrication of constructs with intricate pore geometries, dentinal tubule-like channels, and enamel-mimetic surface textures (Kim et al., 2020). Such resolution is crucial for supporting cellular infiltration, vascularization, and nutrient diffusion within engineered tissues. Improvements in optical systems, photopolymerization chemistries, and slicing algorithms have dramatically accelerated printing speed while maintaining high fidelity. These advances allow the rapid fabrication of patient-specific scaffolds and prototypes, reducing laboratory processing time and improving workflow efficiency. High-resolution platforms are particularly instrumental in engineering periodontal ligament interfaces, root surface geometries, and complex multilayer dental constructs that require precise spatial control.

3.5.4 Multimaterial and multilayer printing techniques

Multimaterial and multilayer bioprinting represent an important evolution in the field, enabling fabrication of heterogeneous structures that emulate the hierarchical organization of natural dental tissues. By depositing multiple materials simultaneously, such as stiff ceramic composites for load-bearing regions and soft, cell-laden hydrogels for regenerative zones, bioprinting systems can create integrated constructs with region-specific mechanical and biological properties (Ozbolat et al., 2017). This approach is particularly advantageous for producing biomimetic, stratified structures. For instance, a dental construct might be printed with a hard, wear-resistant enamel-like outer layer, a more flexible dentin-like sublayer, and a soft, biologically active pulp core. Such gradients closely replicate the functional performance of natural teeth, enhancing durability, shock absorption, and physiological responsiveness. Multilayer printing also facilitates the development of periodontal complexes wherein cementum, ligament, and alveolar bone components are printed in coordinated sequences.

3.6 SUMMARY

This chapter discusses the core principles, material systems, and emerging clinical uses of 3D bioprinting in dentistry. It outlines the biological and procedural constraints of current interventions, emphasizing the need for approaches that support tissue preservation, improve integration, and enable individualized treatment planning. This chapter also examines the key bioprinting technologies, including inkjet bioprinting, SLA, DLP, and multimaterial platforms for their capacity to fabricate high-precision constructs suitable for dental and periodontal applications. It also evaluated major classes of bioinks such as hydrogels, ceramics, and composite systems, highlighting their role in reproducing the structural and functional characteristics of native oral tissues. Consideration was given to scaffold architecture and surface modification strategies, with emphasis on methods that improve cell attachment, promote regeneration, and enhance long-term performance. Recent developments in AI and ML were reviewed as important additions to bioprinting workflows, contributing to greater accuracy, reproducibility, and predictive capability. Applications across prosthodontics, periodontal regeneration, implant design, and orthodontics illustrate the breadth of opportunities for integrating bioprinting technologies into clinical workflows.

REFERENCES

Chen, C., Hou, X., Zhao, Y., & Zhang, Y. (2020). Advances in 3D printing technology in orthodontics: A comprehensive review. *International Journal of Oral Science*, 12(1), 1–9.

Dawood, A., Marti Marti, B., Sauret-Jackson, V., & Darwood, A. (2015). 3D printing in dentistry. *British Dental Journal*, 219(11), 521–529.

Ge, Z., Wang, L., Heng, B. C., Tian, X. F., Lu, K., Fan, V. T. W., Yeo, J. F., & Cao, T. (2009). Proliferation and differentiation of human osteoblasts within 3D printed poly-lactic-co-glycolic acid scaffolds. *Journal of Biomaterials Applications*, 23(6), 533–547.

Han, Y., Xu, J., Chopra, H., Zhang, Z., Dubey, N., Dissanayaka, W. L., Nör, J. E., & Bottino, M. C. (2024). Injectable tissue-specific hydrogel system for pulp-dentin regeneration. *Journal of Dental Research*, 103(4), 398–408.

Kim, J., Kim, S., & Kim, H. W. (2020). Nanoengineered biomaterial approaches for dental tissue regeneration: Progress and challenges. *Journal of Dental Research*, 99(8), 937–946.

Moghaddaszadeh, A., Seddiqi, H., Najmoddin, N., Abbasi Ravasjani, S., & Klein-Nulend, J. (2021). Biomimetic 3D-printed PCL scaffold containing a high concentration carbonated-nanohydroxyapatite with immobilized-collagen for bone tissue engineering: Enhanced bioactivity and physicomechanical characteristics. *Biomedical Materials*, 16(6), 065019.

Murphy, S. V., & Atala, A. (2014). 3D bioprinting of tissues and organs. *Nature Biotechnology*, 32(8), 773–785.

Murphy, S. V., & Atala, A. (2020). Bioprinting for oral and dental tissue engineering. *Journal of Dental Research*, 99(10), 1218–1225.

Nguyen, D., Hägg, A., Forsman, A., Ekholm, J., & Gatenholm, P. (2021). Machine learning in extrusion-based 3D bioprinting: Predicting printing outcomes for bioinks. *ACS Biomaterials Science and Engineering*, 7(8), 3593–3603.

Ong, J. L., Oral, E., & Bertassoni, L. E. (2017). Biomaterials for dental applications: Current trends and future directions. *Dental Materials*, 33(10), 1–10.

Ozbolat, I. T., Hospodiuk, M., & Koc, P. (2017). Multimaterial bioprinting for integrated tissue fabrication. *Trends in Biotechnology*, 35(9), 735–742.

Rasperini, G., Pilipchuk, S. P., Flanagan, C. L., Park, C. H., Pagni, G., Hollister, S. J., & Giannobile, W. V. (2015). 3D-printed bioresorbable scaffold for periodontal repair. *Journal of Dental Research*, 94(9_suppl), 153S–157S.

Santana, L., Menezes, R. M., Lima, L. M., & Menezes, R. R. (2020). Machine learning applied to micro-CT characterization of 3D-printed scaffolds for bone tissue engineering. *Materials Science and Engineering:* C, 109, 110539.

Turkyilmaz, I., & Wilkins, G. N. (2021). 3D printing in dentistry: Exploring the new horizons. *Journal of Dental Sciences*, 16(3), 1037–1043.

Ventola, C. L. (2014). Medical applications for 3D printing: Current and projected uses. *Pharmacy and Therapeutics*, 39(10), 704–711.

Wang, X., Ao, K., Yu, J., & Zhang, X. (2021). Hybrid bioinks for 3D bioprinting in dental tissue regeneration: Enhanced mechanical properties, cell viability, and tissue-specific bioactivity. *Acta Biomaterialia*, 121, 240–256.

Chapter 4

Scaffolds in dental tissue engineering

4.1 INTRODUCTION

Scaffolds constitute a central component of contemporary tissue engineering, functioning as three-dimensional (3D) frameworks that facilitate the restoration and regeneration of damaged or missing tissues. By emulating the architecture and biological functions of the extracellular matrix (ECM), these constructs provide essential structural support while presenting biochemical and biophysical signals that regulate cellular adhesion, proliferation, migration, and differentiation. Within dental tissue engineering, scaffolds underpin regenerative strategies targeting the pulp–dentin complex, periodontal ligament, cementum, and alveolar bone. Their design has advanced substantially in recent years, integrating innovative biomaterials, hierarchical architectures, and precision fabrication technologies to address the distinct mechanical, biological, and spatial demands of dental tissue repair.

The primary role of scaffolds is to establish a permissive microenvironment that supports cellular adhesion, proliferation, and lineage-specific differentiation. By providing spatial organization and biochemical signals, these constructs facilitate the deposition of new tissue matrices while undergoing controlled biodegradation in concert with native tissue regeneration. Scaffold systems may be engineered from natural biomaterials such as collagen or from synthetic polymers including poly(lactic-co-glycolic acid) (PLGA), with hybrid formulations frequently employed to balance biocompatibility, mechanical integrity, and degradation kinetics (Neves et al., 2020; Jazayeri et al., 2020). These materials are often functionalized with growth factors or signaling molecules to modulate cellular behavior, thereby enhancing the regenerative capacity of stem cells incorporated within the scaffold architecture.

In endodontic applications, scaffold-based strategies are particularly critical for the revitalization of the pulp–dentin complex, where regeneration is impeded by limited anatomical space, restricted vascular supply, and the specialized arrangement of resident cell populations. Advances in additive manufacturing, including high-resolution 3D printing, have enabled

DOI: 10.1201/9781003589921-4

the production of patient-specific scaffolds tailored to the geometry and functional needs of individual root canal systems. Furthermore, the integration of scaffold platforms with stem-cell-derived organoid systems has significantly expanded the potential for recapitulating the structural, molecular, and functional characteristics of native dental tissues, marking an important evolution in personalized regenerative endodontics.

4.2 ROLE OF SCAFFOLDS IN SUPPORTING CELLULAR ACTIVITIES AND TISSUE REGENERATION

Scaffolds are indispensable components of dental tissue engineering because of their multifaceted role in regulating cellular behavior and orchestrating tissue regeneration. A fundamental function of these constructs is to provide a substrate that supports cell adhesion, an essential prerequisite for subsequent proliferation, migration, and lineage commitment (Figure 4.1). Through their ECM mimetic properties, scaffolds establish both structural and biochemical signals that facilitate cell–matrix interactions and enhance the regenerative potential of stem cell populations such as dental pulp stem

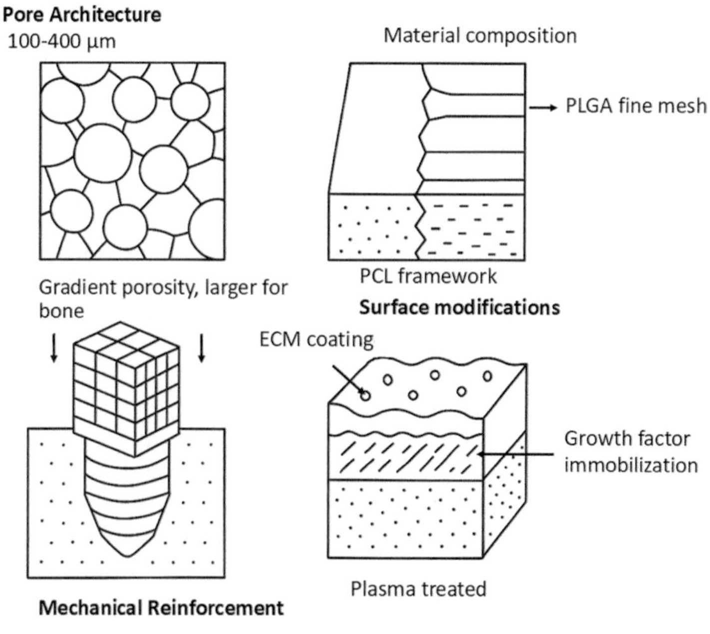

Figure 4.1 Bioinks that are used in dental bioprinting. The diagram categorizes hydrogels, ceramics, and composite systems that are used in dental regeneration. It illustrates their mechanical properties, biological functions, and tissue-specific relevance, including applications in pulp, periodontal ligament, dentin, and alveolar bone engineering.

cells (DPSCs) and stem cells from the apical papilla (SCAP) (Abolhasani et al., 2025; Thirumalaivasan 2025).

Also, scaffolds actively modulate cellular function through the controlled presentation and release of bioactive molecules. Incorporation of growth factors, including transforming growth factor-β (TGF-β) and vascular endothelial growth factor (VEGF), enables spatially and temporally regulated signaling that directs stem cell differentiation toward odontogenic or angiogenic phenotypes, both of which are essential for the reconstitution of the pulp–dentin complex (Jazayeri et al., 2020; Galler et al., 2011). For instance, VEGF drives neovascularization to ensure adequate perfusion of the regenerating tissue, whereas TGF-β promotes the differentiation of progenitor cells into odontoblast-like cells that contribute to reparative dentin formation.

The scaffold architecture further determines the biological success of regeneration. Porous constructs with interconnected micro- and macro-networks enable efficient diffusion of nutrients, gases, and metabolic waste, thereby supporting cell viability within the confined root canal environment. Advances in fabrication technologies, such as electrospinning and additive manufacturing, now permit the precise control of pore size, orientation, and spatial distribution, yielding engineered matrices that more closely replicate the hierarchical organization of the native ECM. Additionally, optimized mechanical properties confer stability to the regenerating tissue, shielding it from functional stresses during early healing.

Scaffolds also function as delivery vehicles for antimicrobial and anti-inflammatory agents, reducing microbial load and modulating the host inflammatory response within the canal. This dual capacity to sustain desirable cellular activities while counteracting pathological conditions positions scaffolds as a central determinant of success in contemporary regenerative endodontic procedures.

4.3 IMPORTANCE OF SCAFFOLDS IN INTEGRATING 3D ORGANOIDS AND STEM CELLS FOR REGENERATIVE ENDODONTICS

The convergence of scaffold technologies with 3D organoids and stem cell-based systems represents one of the most advanced directions in regenerative endodontics, enabling the recreation of the structural and functional intricacies of native dental tissues. Organoids, derived from self-organizing stem cell populations, recapitulate essential features of tissue architecture and cellular heterogeneity. When integrated with biomimetic scaffolds, they are provided with a supportive microenvironment that permits spatial organization, lineage specification, and functional maturation.

Within this integrated platform, scaffolds serve as both a physical matrix and a source of instructive biochemical stimuli. Seeding DPSCs or SCAP onto scaffold substrates, along with defined signaling molecules, enables the generation of engineered pulp–dentin constructs with emerging characteristics of native tissue. The ECM-like properties of the scaffold promote cell adhesion and proliferation, while controlled delivery of morphogens facilitates directed differentiation into odontoblast-like phenotypes responsible for dentin formation (Kim et al., 2018).

A persistent limitation in regenerative endodontics is the recreation of a functional vascular supply as the vitality of the dental pulp is critically dependent on adequate perfusion. Scaffold systems help overcome this constraint by incorporating angiogenic stimuli such as VEGF, which stimulate endothelial cell recruitment and neovascularization within the engineered microenvironment. Emerging fabrication strategies, particularly high-resolution 3D bioprinting, further enable the spatial integration of predesigned vascular channels into scaffold architectures, markedly improving nutrient exchange, oxygenation, and long-term tissue viability.

The scaffold–organoid composite also provides a versatile platform for modeling disease mechanisms and evaluating therapeutic interventions. By generating pathology-specific organoids within scaffold constructs, investigators can examine the interplay between inflammatory mediators, cellular stress responses, and regenerative processes in a controlled 3D context. This approach offers new opportunities for mechanistic discovery and preclinical testing of biomaterials, pharmaceuticals, and biologics intended for clinical translation in regenerative endodontics.

4.4 BIOMATERIALS FOR SCAFFOLD DESIGN

Biomaterials form the foundation of scaffold-based strategies in dental tissue engineering as their physicochemical and biological properties directly determine scaffold performance, influencing cell compatibility, mechanical integrity, and degradation dynamics (Table 4.1). Scaffolds are fabricated from natural, synthetic, or hybrid biomaterials, each offering distinct advantages and limitations. By replicating key features of the ECM, these materials support cell adhesion, proliferation, and differentiation, thereby facilitating the regeneration of dental tissues.

4.4.1 Natural biomaterials

Natural biomaterials, derived from biological sources, are highly valued in dental tissue engineering for their biocompatibility and ability to mimic the ECM. These materials provide an ideal environment for cell attachment, proliferation, and differentiation due to their intrinsic bioactivity. They also contain natural signaling molecules and structural proteins that facilitate tissue repair and regeneration. Among the most widely used natural

Table 4.1 Comparison of natural, synthetic, and hybrid biomaterials for dental scaffolds

Biomaterials	*Examples*	*Advantages*	*Limitations*	*Applications in dental tissue engineering*
Natural	Collagen, gelatin, hyaluronic acid, and decellularized ECM	Biocompatible, mimics native ECM, and promotes cell adhesion	Rapid degradation and variability in properties	Pulp–dentin regeneration and periodontal scaffolds
Synthetic	PLGA, PEG, and PCL	Tunable mechanical properties and controlled degradation	Lacks bioactivity and potential cytotoxicity	Alveolar bone regeneration and scaffolds for implants
Hybrid	Collagen-PLGA, gelatin-PEG, and decellularized ECM–synthetic composites	Combines bioactivity with mechanical strength	Complex fabrication and cost-intensive	Multitissue scaffolds and pulp regeneration

biomaterials in scaffold design are collagen, gelatin, hyaluronic acid, and decellularized tissues.

Collagen, the most abundant protein in the ECM, serves as the foundation for many scaffold designs. Its fibrillar structure closely resembles the natural ECM, promoting cellular adhesion and migration. Collagen scaffolds also support the differentiation of DPSCs and SCAP into odontoblast-like cells, essential for dentin regeneration. Studies have shown that collagen-based scaffolds enhance the formation of reparative dentin when combined with bioactive molecules like TGF-β (Galler et al., 2011).

Gelatin, a hydrolyzed form of collagen, retains the bioactive properties of its precursor while offering improved solubility and processability. Gelatin-based scaffolds are often cross-linked to enhance their mechanical strength and degradation rates. These scaffolds have been successfully used in pulp–dentin complex regeneration, supporting angiogenesis and the formation of new blood vessels, which are critical for pulp revitalization.

Hyaluronic acid, a glycosaminoglycan found in connective tissues, is another promising natural biomaterial. It provides hydration and facilitates cell migration, making it suitable for applications requiring soft-tissue regeneration. Modified hyaluronic acid scaffolds have shown potential in delivering growth factors and stem cells for pulp regeneration.

Decellularized tissues, such as decellularized dental pulp, provide natural scaffolds that retain the ECM's structural integrity and bioactivity. These scaffolds are obtained by removing cellular components while preserving proteins, glycoproteins, and signaling molecules. Decellularized pulp scaffolds have been shown to enhance cellular repopulation and support the formation of vascularized pulp-like tissue (Neves et al., 2020). Despite their advantages, natural biomaterials often face challenges, including variability in mechanical properties, rapid degradation, and potential immunogenicity. These limitations have spurred interest in synthetic and hybrid biomaterials that address these shortcomings while retaining the bioactivity of natural materials.

4.4.2 Synthetic biomaterials

Synthetic biomaterials offer a high degree of tunability, allowing for the customization of mechanical properties, degradation rates, and bioactivity. They are manufactured through chemical processes, which ensure consistency and reproducibility. Synthetic biomaterials like PLGA, polyethylene glycol (PEG), and polycaprolactone (PCL) are widely used in dental tissue engineering.

PLGA is a biodegradable polymer approved by the FDA for various medical applications. Its degradation rate can be adjusted by altering the ratio of lactic acid to glycolic acid, making it suitable for different tissue engineering needs. PLGA scaffolds have been used to deliver growth factors such as VEGF and bone morphogenetic proteins (BMPs), enhancing angiogenesis and bone regeneration (Jazayeri et al., 2020). In dental tissue engineering, PLGA scaffolds provide structural support for pulp–dentin complex regeneration.

PEG is a hydrophilic polymer known for its biocompatibility and resistance to protein adsorption. PEG-based hydrogels are commonly used as scaffolds in regenerative endodontics due to their ability to create a hydrated environment that mimics natural tissues. PEG can be functionalized with bioactive molecules, making it a versatile option for scaffold design. PCL is a semi-crystalline polymer with excellent mechanical properties and a slow degradation rate. These characteristics make it suitable for applications requiring long-term structural support, such as alveolar bone regeneration. PCL scaffolds have been used in combination with stem cells and growth factors to promote osteogenesis and dentinogenesis. Although synthetic biomaterials excel in mechanical stability and tunability, they lack the inherent bioactivity of natural materials. Efforts to enhance their performance include incorporating bioactive molecules and combining them with natural biomaterials to create hybrid scaffolds.

4.4.3 Hybrid biomaterials

Hybrid biomaterials combine the strengths of natural and synthetic components, offering a balanced and highly adaptable strategy for scaffold design. By integrating the intrinsic bioactivity of natural polymers with mechanical stability, controlled degradation, and tunability of synthetic materials, hybrid scaffolds effectively address limitations associated with using either class alone. Collagen–PLGA scaffolds exemplify this approach as the collagen fraction provides a biologically favorable interface that supports cellular adhesion and proliferation, while PLGA contributes structural stability and predictable biodegradation, resulting in enhanced cellular responses and improved pulp–dentin complex regeneration in preclinical models (Kim et al., 2018). Similarly, gelatin–PEG hydrogels merge the biological functionality of gelatin with the physicochemical stability and hydration properties of PEG, creating versatile matrices that can functionalize growth factors to promote both odontogenic and angiogenic differentiation. Decellularized ECM–synthetic composites further extend this concept by incorporating native ECM components into synthetic backbones, yielding scaffolds that retain natural bioactivity while benefiting from the durability and processing advantages of synthetic polymers, with promising results in regenerating complex tissues such as the pulp–dentin complex (Neves et al., 2020). Together, these hybrid systems represent a forward-looking approach in scaffold engineering, offering customizable platforms tailored to the specific structural and biological demands of different dental tissues and thereby improving regenerative outcomes.

4.5 SCAFFOLDS AND STEM CELL INTEGRATION IN DENTAL TISSUE ENGINEERING

Building on the advantages of these biomaterial systems, scaffolds also serve as critical regulators of stem cell behavior in dental tissue engineering, enabling the effective application of DPSCs, SCAP, and other mesenchymal stem cells (MSCs). Acting as synthetic analogs of the ECM, scaffolds provide the architectural and biochemical context necessary for stem cell survival, proliferation, and differentiation. DPSCs, known for their proliferative capacity and ability to differentiate into odontoblast-like cells, rely on scaffold-derived stimuli to adhere, migrate, and initiate dentin matrix deposition. Rosales-Ibáñez et al. (2021) demonstrated that 3D-printed PCL scaffolds readily support human DPSC attachment and proliferation, with good viability and mineralization, highlighting their utility for bone/dentin regeneration. Gao et al. (2025) similarly emphasize DPSCs as the preferred seeding cells for pulp regeneration and note that scaffolds can offer a 3D architecture to support the regenerative microenvironment and sustain stem cell viability and functionality. Collagen-based scaffolds have proven highly effective due to their close resemblance to native pulp ECM, supporting stemness maintenance and promoting odontoblastic differentiation (Neves et al., 2020). SCAP, which exhibit strong odontogenic potential (Huang et al., 2025) and play a pivotal role in root development and apexogenesis, similarly depend on scaffold structures to populate damaged or necrotic regions of the canal system and maintain regenerative functionality. Additional MSCs such as periodontal ligament stem cells and induced pluripotent stem cells also benefit from scaffold integration as scaffolds act as carriers that ensure cellular retention at target sites, prevent cell loss, and facilitate localized differentiation. Through these combined mechanical and biochemical roles, scaffolds become indispensable in supporting the structural integrity of engineered tissues while simultaneously guiding cellular activities critical for effective regeneration.

4.6 ENHANCEMENT OF CELLULAR PROLIFERATION AND DIFFERENTIATION THROUGH SCAFFOLD DESIGN

This interplay between scaffold design and stem cell behavior is further refined through carefully engineered scaffold properties that enhance cellular proliferation and differentiation. Porosity remains a core design parameter as interconnected pore networks facilitate nutrient and oxygen exchange, metabolic waste removal, and uniform cell migration throughout the scaffold. Nanofibrous architectures produced via electrospinning are especially effective in replicating the fibrous structure of the native ECM, providing an environment that closely resembles natural dental tissues and encourages robust cell adhesion and proliferation (Galler et al., 2011). Surface modification further strengthens scaffold–cell interactions by incorporating bioactive sequences such as RGD motifs that enhance integrin-mediated adhesion and migration, while nanoscale surface topographies modulate the cellular morphology and cytoskeletal organization through mechano-transduction pathways, ultimately guiding odontogenic differentiation.

Material selection also remains essential as biodegradable polymers like PLGA and natural components like collagen support cellular activity yet differ in mechanical behavior and degradation rates. Hybrid materials thus offer a strategic solution by combining bioactivity with mechanical resilience. In parallel, advanced scaffold designs are increasingly incorporating stimuli-responsive features that enable the controlled release of bioactive molecules in response to environmental signals such as pH or temperature, thereby promoting lineage-specific differentiation of DPSCs and SCAP and facilitating reparative dentin formation. Through the optimization of scaffold architecture, chemistry, and functionalization, researchers continue to refine these platforms to more effectively enhance stem cell proliferation and differentiation, driving progress toward more predictable and successful regenerative therapies.

4.7 USE OF SCAFFOLDS IN CONJUNCTION WITH GROWTH FACTORS

The integration of growth factors into scaffolds is a crucial strategy for modulating stem cell behavior and enhancing regenerative outcomes in dental tissue engineering. Growth factors such as TGF-β, VEGF, and BMPs regulate odontogenic and angiogenic pathways that are fundamental to dental tissue regeneration (Table 4.2). When incorporated into scaffold matrices, these signaling molecules create a bioactive microenvironment that directs cellular activities in a spatially and temporally controlled manner.

TGF-β is central to the differentiation of DPSCs and SCAP into odontoblast-like phenotypes. Scaffold-mediated delivery of TGF-β upregulates key odontogenic markers including dentin sialophosphoprotein and dentin matrix protein-1, both essential for dentin matrix deposition. Controlled-release systems ensure prolonged and localized availability of TGF-β, improving its bioactivity while reducing systemic dispersal and off-target effects (Jazayeri et al., 2020). This sustained presentation enhances the formation of reparative dentin and supports the maturation of newly differentiated odontoblast-like cells.

VEGF, in contrast, is indispensable for angiogenesis and the establishment of functional vascular networks within regenerating tissues. Scaffolds enriched with VEGF stimulate endothelial cell recruitment and capillary formation, thereby improving oxygenation and nutrient transport within the engineered microenvironment. This vascularization is vital for the survival, proliferation, and differentiation of DPSCs and other stem cell populations.

Table 4.2 Integration of growth factors into scaffolds for regenerative endodontics

Growth factor	*Function*	*Role in regeneration*	*Application in dental tissue engineering*
Transforming growth factor-beta (TGF-β)	Regulates stem cell differentiation	Enhances odontoblast formation	Dentin–pulp regeneration
Bone morphogenetic proteins (BMPs)	Induces bone and dentin formation	Supports osteogenesis and dentinogenesis	Alveolar bone regeneration and root repair
Vascular endothelial growth factor (VEGF)	Stimulates blood vessel formation	Enhances angiogenesis in scaffolds	Vascularized pulp regeneration
Platelet-derived growth factor (PDGF)	Promotes cell proliferation	Supports periodontal ligament repair	Periodontal tissue engineering
Fibroblast growth factor (FGF)	Supports fibroblast and endothelial cell activity	Enhances soft-tissue regeneration	Gingival and connective tissue repair

Empirical studies have demonstrated that VEGF-loaded scaffolds not only enhance neovascularization but also accelerate the regeneration of vascularized pulp-like tissue (Neves et al., 2020).

BMPs contribute significantly to osteogenic differentiation and mineralized tissue formation, making them particularly useful in applications targeting alveolar bone regeneration. Scaffolds incorporating BMPs have shown improved mineral deposition and enhanced bone formation, thereby complementing broader strategies in dental tissue engineering aimed at restoring both soft and hard tissues. Umapathy et al. (2025) reviewed the roles of key factors, BMP-2 and BMP-7, thatinduce odontogenic and osteogenic differentiation of dental stem cells, TGF-β that regulates dentin matrix secretion, and VEGF that is essential for neovascularization in pulp regeneration.

Together, the combination of scaffolds and growth factors enables precise control over cellular activities, facilitating predictable and effective regenerative outcomes. Continued advances in controlled-release systems and scaffold functionalization have refined the delivery of growth factors, maximizing their therapeutic potential and supporting the development of next-generation regenerative endodontic therapies.

4.8 ADVANCES IN INTEGRATING SCAFFOLDS WITH 3D ORGANOIDS

The integration of scaffolds with 3D organoids represents a major advancement in efforts to replicate the structural and functional complexity of native dental tissues. Organoids, generated from stem cell populations, are self-organizing systems that recapitulate key aspects of the tissue architecture and behavior. When combined with appropriately engineered scaffolds, these organoids receive the physical support and biochemical signals necessary for sustained growth, differentiation, and functional maturation, thereby enhancing their applicability in dental tissue engineering.

Scaffolds significantly improve organoid development by establishing a 3D microenvironment conducive to cell–cell and cell–matrix interactions. Collagen-based constructs, for example, have been successfully seeded with organoids derived from DPSCs, enabling the formation of engineered pulp–dentin-like tissues that closely mirror native structures in terms of cellular composition and ECM organization (Kim et al., 2018). This biomimicry is critical for achieving physiologically relevant models and improving translational potential.

A persistent limitation in organoid-based regeneration is the establishment of adequate vascularization. Scaffolds help address this challenge through the incorporation of angiogenic molecules such as VEGF and, increasingly, through bio-fabricated vascular networks generated using advanced 3D bioprinting techniques. These vascularized scaffolds promote sustained organoid viability, enhance oxygen and nutrient delivery, and support long-term functionality, all of which are essential for successful regenerative applications.

Beyond their therapeutic potential, scaffold–organoid constructs offer powerful *in vitro* platforms for studying dental disease mechanisms and evaluating novel therapeutics. By generating disease-specific organoids within scaffold environments, researchers have modeled conditions such as pulpitis and analyzed complex interactions between inflammatory pathways, cellular responses, and regeneration strategies. Together, the integration of scaffolds with organoid systems marks a paradigm shift in dental tissue engineering, expanding the possibilities for regenerative therapies while providing robust tools for mechanistic research and preclinical testing.

4.9 FABRICATION TECHNIQUES FOR SCAFFOLDS IN DENTAL TISSUE ENGINEERING

Fabrication techniques constitute a critical foundation in scaffold engineering for dental tissue regeneration as they directly influence the resultant scaffold architecture, mechanical properties, and biological performance (Table 4.3). Through these methods, it is possible to construct matrices that emulate the ECM, support essential cellular behaviors, and incorporate bioactive components to direct tissue repair. Among the diverse approaches available, there are three techniques—3D printing, electrospinning, and decellularization. They have emerged as central to the development of scaffolds tailored for regenerative endodontic applications (Figure 4.2).

Table 4.3 Scaffold fabrication techniques in dental tissue engineering

Fabrication technique	*Mechanism*	*Advantages*	*Limitations*	*Example applications*
3D printing	Layer-by-layer deposition of biomaterials	Customizable and high precision	High cost and material limitations	Patient-specific pulp–dentin scaffolds
Electrospinning	High-voltage fiber deposition	Nanofibrous ECM-like structure	Limited 3D control	Dentin regeneration scaffolds
Decellularization	Removal of cellular components from tissues	Retains native ECM composition	Variability in outcomes	Decellularized pulp scaffolds

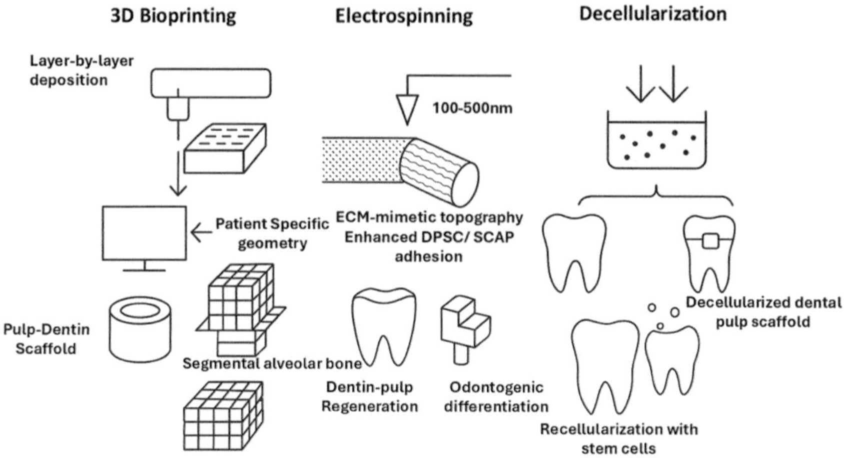

Figure 4.2 Comparison of major scaffold fabrication techniques that are used in dental tissue engineering. The figure contrasts 3D printing, electrospinning, and decellularization based on the architectural output, biomaterial compatibility, biological features, and regenerative applications in pulp–dentin complex, periodontal tissues, and alveolar bone.

4.9.1 3D printing for creating complex geometries and patient-specific scaffolds

3D printing, or additive manufacturing, has emerged as a transformative fabrication strategy in scaffold engineering, offering precise control over architectural parameters, material composition, and functional attributes. By constructing structures layer by layer from digital designs, this technique enables the production of scaffolds with complex geometries that can be tailored to the specific structural and biological requirements of dental tissue regeneration.

A major advantage of 3D printing is its capacity to generate patient-specific scaffolds. Using computed tomography or magnetic resonance imaging datasets, clinicians can develop high-fidelity anatomical models and fabricate scaffolds that conform precisely to individual defect morphologies. Such customization enhances integration with host tissues, reduces procedural complications, and improves the predictability of regenerative outcomes (Kim et al., 2018). In the context of pulp–dentin regeneration, 3D-printed constructs can recapitulate the intricate morphology of the pulp chamber and root canal system, facilitating optimal interaction with resident tissues and cell populations.

The technique further allows for spatial integration of multiple materials within a single construct, enabling the development of hybrid scaffolds with controlled gradients in biological and mechanical properties.

This capability is particularly useful for mimicking the heterogeneous composition of dental tissues. For example, scaffolds combining bioactive phases such as collagen with mechanically resilient polymers like PLGA have demonstrated improved cellular adhesion while maintaining structural stability throughout the regenerative process.

An advanced extension of 3D printing is bioprinting, in which living cells, biomolecules, and bioactive materials are incorporated directly into the fabrication process. This approach enables the generation of constructs that not only replicate the architecture of native tissues but also exhibit intrinsic biological functionality. Experimental studies have shown that bioprinted scaffolds containing DPSCs and VEGF promote angiogenesis and support the formation of pulp-like tissue structures (Jazayeri et al., 2020). Despite these advantages, several limitations persist, including the high cost of printing equipment and biomaterials, constraints imposed by the printability of certain polymers, and the need for post-processing to improve mechanical robustness or biological performance. Ongoing advances in printing resolution, bioink development, and multimaterial printing platforms are continually addressing these challenges, solidifying 3D printing as an increasingly practical and impactful technique for scaffold fabrication in dental tissue engineering.

4.9.2 Electrospinning for producing nanofibrous ECM-like structures

Electrospinning is an extensively employed technique for fabricating nanofibrous scaffolds that replicate the fibrous architecture of the natural ECM. In this process, a high-voltage electric field is applied to a polymer solution or melt, generating ultrafine fibers that are deposited as a nonwoven mat. The resulting nanofibrous network possesses a high surface area and porosity, features that significantly enhance cell adhesion, proliferation, and subsequent tissue-specific responses.

The nanoscale topography of electrospun scaffolds closely parallels the structural characteristics of the native ECM, creating a microenvironment favorable for stem cell activities. These scaffolds effectively support the attachment and migration of DPSCs and SCAP, promoting their differentiation into odontoblast-like phenotypes. Experimental studies have shown that electrospun matrices enhance odontogenic differentiation and contribute to reparative dentin formation (Galler et al., 2011). A major advantage of electrospinning is its compatibility with a broad spectrum of polymers, including natural materials such as collagen and synthetic polymers such as PCL. Hybrid nanofibrous constructs combining these materials harness the bioactivity of natural components and the mechanical resilience of synthetic polymers. Collagen–PCL scaffolds, for example, have demonstrated strong potential in promoting angiogenesis and dentinogenesis, processes essential for regenerating the pulp–dentin complex.

Functionalization of electrospun scaffolds with bioactive signaling molecules further amplifies their regenerative capability. Incorporation of TGF-β or platelet-derived growth factor into nanofibrous constructs has been shown to enhance odontogenic differentiation and vascularization, improving outcomes in dentin regeneration. In addition, electrospinning enables the fabrication of multilayered scaffolds containing distinct functional zones, which can mimic the hierarchical organization of dental tissues. Despite these advantages, electrospinning alone is limited in its capacity to produce 3D constructs with complex macroscopic geometries. Integrating electrospinning with complementary fabrication methods, such as 3D printing, offers a promising hybrid approach that merges the ECM-like characteristics of electrospun nanofibers with the structural complexity achievable through additive manufacturing, thereby broadening the scope of scaffold design for dental tissue engineering.

4.9.3 Decellularization for preserving the native ECM architecture

Decellularization is a fabrication strategy that removes cellular components from tissues while preserving the structural and biochemical characteristics of the ECM. This technique yields biologically derived scaffolds that maintain the native tissue's architecture and intrinsic bioactive molecules, making them highly suitable for tissue-specific regeneration. In dental tissue engineering, decellularized matrices have attracted considerable interest, particularly for regenerating the pulp–dentin complex. Decellularized human dental pulp, for example, provides a naturally derived framework that supports cell adhesion, proliferation, and differentiation and retains key ECM constituents such as collagen, proteoglycans, and glycoproteins, all of which contribute to a microenvironment conducive to repair and regeneration (Neves et al., 2020). The decellularization process commonly employs chemical detergents, enzymatic treatments, or physical modalities to eliminate the cellular material while minimizing disruption to the ECM. Achieving complete removal of immunogenic components alongside preservation of structural and biochemical integrity remains a central objective, and refinements in decellularization protocols have increasingly succeeded in balancing these requirements to produce scaffolds with improved regenerative potential.

When seeded with stem cells such as DPSCs or SCAP, decellularized scaffolds effectively support odontoblastic differentiation and promote reparative dentin formation. These matrices also encourage vascularization, a critical determinant of long-term tissue viability and function. Further functionalization with growth factors can augment the inherent bioactivity of decellularized scaffolds, accelerating regenerative processes. Despite their advantages, several challenges remain in translating decellularized scaffolds to clinical practice. Scalability and standardization continue to be limiting factors as the process is labor- and resource-intensive, and variability among tissue sources can lead to inconsistencies in scaffold properties. Addressing these issues will be essential for enabling the broader clinical application of decellularized scaffolds in regenerative endodontics.

4.10 SUMMARY

Scaffolds have emerged as central elements in contemporary dental tissue engineering, providing the structural framework, biochemical signals, and dynamic microenvironment required to support the regeneration of complex dental tissues. Advances in biomaterial science have enabled the development of natural, synthetic, and hybrid scaffold systems that more accurately recapitulate the ECM and modulate stem cell behavior. These engineered platforms enhance the adhesion, proliferation, and lineage-specific differentiation of DPSCs, SCAP, and other MSC populations, thereby facilitating the formation of dentin, pulp tissue, periodontal structures, and alveolar bone. The integration of growth factors, bioactive molecules, and stem cells has further expanded the functional capacity of scaffolds, enabling precise control over odontogenic, angiogenic, and osteogenic pathways critical for successful regeneration. Parallel progress in fabrication technologies such as 3D printing, electrospinning, and decellularization has allowed the creation of architecturally and biologically sophisticated scaffolds that mimic native tissue environments with increasing fidelity. These advances have made it possible to tailor scaffold properties at macro-, micro-, and nanoscale levels; enhance vascularization; and incorporate patient-specific structural features. Emerging approaches that combine scaffold systems with organoid and bioprinting technologies represent an important evolution in the field, offering unprecedented opportunities to recapitulate native tissue complexity, model disease mechanisms *in vitro*, and advance personalized regenerative endodontic therapies. While challenges remain, including standardization of biomaterial sources, optimization of controlled-release systems, and the translation of laboratory protocols into clinically scalable workflows, the trajectory of current research strongly supports the continued integration of biomaterials science, stem cell biology, and advanced fabrication techniques.

REFERENCES

Abolhasani, S., Ahmadi, Y., Rostami, Y., Baravar, E., & Fattahi, D. (2025, August). Biomaterials in tissue repair and regeneration: Key insights from extracellular matrix biology. *Frontiers in Medical Technology*, 7, 1565810. https://doi.org/10.3389/fmedt.2025.1565810

Galler, K. M., D'Souza, R. N., Federlin, M., Cavender, A. C., & Hartgerink, J. D. (2011). Scaffolds for dental pulp tissue engineering. *Advances in Dental Research*, 23(3), 333–339.

Gao, J., Wang, Y., Zhang, T., Qu, J., Liu, Q., Chen, Y., Xu, B., & Shen, J. (2025, July). Dental pulp stem cells conditioned medium-functionalized microspheres for endodontic regeneration. *Frontiers in Cell and Developmental Biology*, 13, 1627220. https://doi.org/10.3389/fcell.2025.1627220

Huang, M., Dissanayaka, W. L., & Yiu, C. K. Y. (2025). Exploring the potential of stem cells from the apical papilla (SCAPs) in regenerative medicine: Advantages, applications, challenges and opportunities. *Stem Cell Research & Therapy*, 16, 626. https://doi.org/10.1186/s13287-025-04705-8

Jazayeri, H. E., Lee, S.-M., Kuhn, L., Fahimipour, F., Tahriri, M., & Tayebi, L. (2020). Polymeric scaffolds for dental pulp tissue engineering: A review. School of Dentistry Faculty Research and Publications. 429. https://epublications.marquette.edu/dentistry_fac/429.

Kim, S. G., Malek, M., Sigurdsson, A., Lin, L. M., & Kahler, B. (2018). Regenerative endodontics: a comprehensive review. *International Endodontic Journal*, 51, 1367–1388.

Neves, V. C., Babb, R., & Sharpe, P. T. (2020). Decellularized human dental pulp as a natural scaffold for regenerative endodontics. *Journal of Endodontics*, 46(12), 1640–1647.

Rosales-Ibáñez, R., Manríquez, J. M., Martínez-González, R., Aguilera-Camacho, Y., & Moreno-Flores, J. M. (2021). Assessment of a PCL-3D printing–dental pulp stem cells triplet for bone engineering: An in vitro study. *Polymers*, 13(7), 1154. https://doi.org/10.3390/polym13071154

Thirumalaivasan, N. (2025). Collagen-composite scaffolds for alveolar bone and dental tissue regeneration: Advances in material development and clinical applications — A narrative review. *Dentistry Journal*, 13(9), 396. https://doi.org/10.3390/dj13090396

Umapathy, V. R., Natarajan, P. M., & Swamikannu, B. (2025). Regenerative strategies in dentistry: Harnessing stem cells, biomaterials and bioactive materials for tissue repair. *Biomolecules*, 15(4), 546.

Chapter 5

Stem cells in regenerative endodontics

5.1 INTRODUCTION

Regenerative endodontics has progressed rapidly over the past two decades and now forms a central component of biologically based dental therapeutics. The field departs from conventional endodontic practice by aiming not only to eliminate infection but also to restore the lost biological functions of the pulp–dentin complex. This shift has been driven largely by advances in stem cell biology. Because of their capacity for self-renewal, multilineage differentiation, and secretion of trophic factors, dental stem cells have become key candidates for rebuilding tissues compromised by caries, trauma, or persistent inflammation. In traditional root canal therapy, removal of the necrotic or infected pulp allows the tooth to remain in function, yet the procedure renders the tooth devoid of vascular, immunologic, and sensory mechanisms that are integral to its physiology. The resulting structure is mechanically preserved but biologically inactive, which may influence its long-term resilience and susceptibility to fracture. These limitations have prompted increasing interest in approaches that aim to restore a living tissue within the root canal space.

Current research demonstrates that several populations of dental stem cells including dental pulp stem cells (DPSCs), stem cells from the apical papilla (SCAP), and periodontal ligament stem cells (PDLSCs) possess the ability to generate odontoblast-like cells, promote neovascularization, and support neural repair. Their secretory activity further contributes to immunomodulation and matrix remodeling, both of which are essential for creating a microenvironment conducive to tissue renewal. By drawing on principles from developmental biology, tissue engineering, and biomaterials science, regenerative endodontics now seek to recreate the structural organization and functional attributes of the native pulp–dentin complex rather than merely stabilizing the tooth. This chapter presents the ongoing efforts to integrate stem cell biology with engineered scaffolds, bioactive signaling molecules, and emerging biomimetic systems.

DOI: 10.1201/9781003589921-5

5.2 STEM CELL SOURCES IN REGENERATIVE ENDODONTICS

The development of regenerative endodontic therapies is closely linked to the availability of well-characterized stem cell populations capable of reconstituting the cellular and extracellular architecture of the pulp–dentin complex. Dental tissues contain several stem cell niches that are both accessible and biologically active, making them particularly suitable for translational applications. These stem cell populations differ in origin, proliferative capacity, differentiation profile, and response to microenvironmental cues, which influences their suitability for specific regenerative strategies. Table 5.1 provides an overview of the principal dental stem cell types currently investigated in this field (Figure 5.1). The following section discusses each source in detail, describing established approaches for their isolation, the defining features of their phenotype and growth behavior, and their documented contributions to pulp regeneration and broader dental tissue repair.

5.2.1 Dental pulp stem cells

DPSCs represent one of the most widely studied mesenchymal stem cell populations in regenerative endodontics. First described by Gronthos and colleagues in (2000), DPSCs have attracted considerable attention because they are readily obtainable from extracted permanent teeth and display strong proliferative and differentiation abilities. These properties, combined with their capacity to contribute to both hard- and soft-tissue formation, position DPSCs as a central component of current regenerative strategies aimed

Table 5.1 Dental stem cells in regenerative endodontics

Stem cells	*Source*	*Differentiation potential*	*Applications in regenerative endodontics*
Dental pulp stem cells (DPSCs)	Dental pulp of permanent teeth	Odontoblasts, osteoblasts, and chondrocytes	Pulp–dentin complex regeneration, and bioengineered teeth
Stem cells from the apical papilla (SCAP)	Apical papilla of immature teeth	Odontoblast-like cells and cementoblasts	Root development and apexogenesis
Periodontal ligament stem cells (PDLSCs)	Periodontal ligament	Cementoblasts, osteoblasts, and fibroblasts	Periodontal repair and cementum regeneration
Dental follicle progenitor cells (DFPCs)	Dental follicle of developing teeth	Cementoblasts, osteoblasts, and fibroblasts	Periodontal and alveolar bone regeneration
Gingival mesenchymal stem cells (GMSCs)	Gingival connective tissue	Osteoblasts, chondrocytes, and adipocytes	Gingival and soft tissue repair and immunomodulation

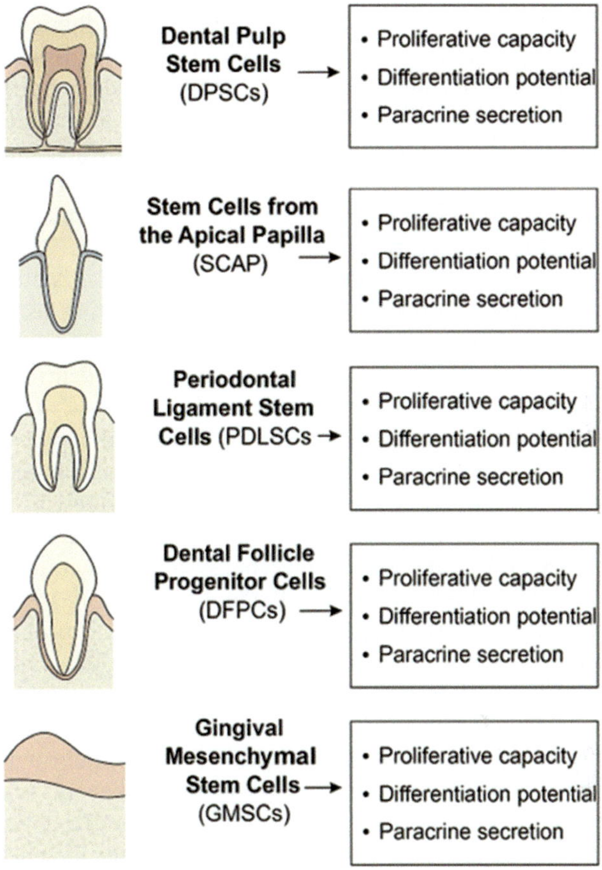

Figure 5.1 Principal sources of dental-derived stem cells and their biological properties. The figure highlights the anatomical origins and functional attributes of dental pulp stem cells, stem cells from the apical papilla, periodontal ligament stem cells, dental follicle progenitor cells, and gingival mesenchymal stem cells.

at restoring the biological function of the pulp–dentin complex. They are isolated from the pulp tissue of extracted teeth, most commonly third molars or premolars removed for orthodontic purposes. Isolation typically involves enzymatic digestion with collagenase and dispase to dissociate the pulp or explant culture techniques that allow cells to migrate from tissue fragments. Once expanded, DPSCs are identified by a characteristic mesenchymal phenotype, expressing markers such as CD73, CD90, and CD105, while lacking hematopoietic markers including CD34 and CD45. Their clonogenicity and reproducible differentiation profile further confirm their identity.

A prominent feature of DPSCs is their robust proliferative capacity, enabling the expansion of clinically relevant cell numbers from small tissue samples. Their multipotent nature allows differentiation into odontoblast-like cells, osteoblasts, chondrocytes, and adipocytes under controlled conditions. Of particular relevance to endodontics is their ability to form dentin-like structures and generate pulp-like tissue that exhibits vascular and neural components. In addition to direct differentiation, DPSCs secrete a range of bioactive molecules such as vascular endothelial growth factor (VEGF) and nerve growth factor, which support angiogenesis, neurogenesis, and modulation of inflammatory responses. These paracrine interactions play a critical role in shaping a microenvironment conducive to tissue regeneration.

The contribution of DPSCs to regenerative endodontics is most evident in experimental and translational models aimed at revitalizing necrotic or damaged pulpal tissue. When delivered into the canal space, DPSCs can differentiate toward an odontoblastic phenotype and deposit new dentin matrix along root walls. At the same time, they facilitate the formation of vascularized and innervated pulp-like tissue, thereby restoring biological activity rather than merely filling the canal space with inert material. These outcomes underscore the importance of DPSCs in strategies that seek to restore normal pulp physiology and enhance long-term tooth survival. They have also been integrated into a wide range of tissue engineering systems that combine stem cells with biomaterial scaffolds and defined signaling molecules. Biodegradable scaffolds serve as templates that support cell attachment, proliferation, and matrix deposition, while recapitulating aspects of the extracellular matrix (ECM). The addition of growth factors such as bone morphogenetic proteins (BMPs) or transforming growth factor beta (TGF-β) can direct DPSC differentiation toward odontoblastic or osteogenic lineages, improving the organization and functionality of the regenerated tissue. Beyond scaffold-based applications, DPSCs have been used in experimental models of bioengineered teeth, where their interaction with epithelial and other mesenchymal stem cell populations has yielded tooth-like structures *in vivo*, illustrating their broader relevance to craniofacial regeneration.

Despite these advantages, several challenges remain before DPSCs can be widely adopted in clinical practice. Pulp tissue can only be harvested through tooth extraction, limiting availability and raising ethical considerations. The biological quality of DPSCs is influenced by donor variables such as age, oral health status, and tooth type, which can affect proliferative capacity and differentiation potential. A further challenge is the lack of standardization across laboratories in isolation, expansion, and delivery protocols, which complicates comparisons across studies and hinders clinical translation. Rigorous long-term studies are required to evaluate the safety, predictability, and durability of DPSC-based therapies in humans.

5.2.2 Stem cells from apical papilla

SCAP constitute a distinct mesenchymal stem cell population derived from the apical papilla, a transient tissue present at the apex of developing permanent teeth. Since their initial characterization, SCAP have become a central focus in regenerative endodontics because of their essential role in root formation, dentinogenesis, and their capacity to support tissue regeneration in immature teeth. Their availability only during the developmental phase gives them a unique biological profile and sets them apart from other dental stem cell sources. They are typically harvested from immature permanent teeth extracted for orthodontic or medical reasons. Isolation generally involves enzymatic digestion of apical papilla tissue using collagenase and dispase, although explant culture methods remain a viable alternative for expanding cell populations. Once isolated, SCAP exhibit a characteristic mesenchymal phenotype, expressing markers such as STRO-1 and CD146, while demonstrating the capacity to differentiate into odontoblast-like cells, osteoblasts, and adipocytes. Their ability to generate both odontogenic and nonodontogenic lineages underscores their functional versatility and relevance to dental tissue regeneration.

Biologically, SCAP possess several properties that distinguish them from other dental stem cell populations. Their proliferative capacity is markedly higher than that observed in DPSCs, enabling efficient expansion even from relatively small volumes of apical tissue. SCAP also exhibit strong paracrine activity, secreting bioactive molecules including VEGF and BMPs. These factors contribute to angiogenic, neurogenic, and tissue remodeling responses, all of which are essential for achieving predictable and functional regeneration in endodontic applications. The role of SCAP in regenerative endodontics is closely linked to their involvement in continued root development and pulp–dentin regeneration. SCAP can differentiate into odontoblast-like cells that produce dentin along the root canal walls, thereby contributing to the structural restoration of teeth with compromised pulp tissue. Their interaction with Hertwig's epithelial root sheath supports the elongation and maturation of the developing root, a process that is particularly important in managing necrotic immature teeth where conventional endodontic procedures often fail to promote root maturation. Recent studies have further demonstrated that SCAP respond dynamically to exogenous biological signals. For example, the antimicrobial peptide LL-37 enhances SCAP migration and odontogenic differentiation through modulation of Akt/Wnt/β-catenin signaling pathways (Huang et al., 2020). This responsiveness to defined molecular stimuli suggests the possibility of refining regenerative protocols by combining SCAP with targeted biological agents. In addition, SCAP integrate effectively with engineered biomaterials, including three-dimensional (3D) scaffolds that replicate ECM features. These scaffolds provide structural support, guide spatial organization, and promote the formation of tissue-like constructs, reinforcing the suitability of SCAP for tissue engineering applications.

Despite their considerable promise, several challenges must be addressed before SCAP-based therapies can be adopted widely in clinical practice. Their availability is limited to early stages of tooth development, and donor variability may influence the yield and quality of isolated cells. Furthermore, the absence of standardized protocols for their isolation, expansion, and clinical delivery hampers cross-study comparisons and delays translation to routine care. Long-term *in vivo* studies remain essential to assess the durability, safety, and functional performance of SCAP-mediated regeneration across different patient populations.

5.2.3 Periodontal ligament stem cells

PDLSCs constitute a well-defined mesenchymal stem cell population located within the periodontal ligament, the fibrous connective tissue that anchors the tooth to the alveolar bone. Since their identification by Seo et al. (2004), PDLSCs have become central to research in dental tissue engineering because of their capacity to contribute to the regeneration of both hard and soft periodontal components. Their biological versatility makes them highly relevant not only to periodontal repair but also to endodontic regeneration, particularly in complex endodontic–periodontal lesions. They are typically isolated from the periodontal ligament of extracted premolars or third molars. Isolation involves enzymatic digestion with collagenase and dispase to release cells from the ligament matrix, followed by expansion under standard culture conditions. Once obtained, PDLSCs exhibit a characteristic mesenchymal phenotype, expressing markers such as CD73, CD90, and CD105, while lacking hematopoietic markers including CD34 and CD45. Their clonogenic growth and reproducible ability to differentiate into multiple lineages confirm their identity as bona fide mesenchymal stem cells. Several biological properties support the therapeutic relevance of PDLSCs. These cells display a strong proliferative capacity that facilitates the generation of sufficient cell numbers for clinical and experimental applications. PDLSCs are also multipotent, capable of differentiating into cementoblasts, osteoblasts, fibroblasts, and adipocytes under defined inductive conditions. Their ability to form cementoblast-like cells is particularly important as cementum regeneration is essential for re-establishing a functional attachment apparatus. In addition to direct differentiation, PDLSCs secrete a wide range of regulatory molecules including VEGF and TGF-β, which contribute to angiogenesis, osteogenesis, and wound healing. Although best known for their role in periodontal regeneration, PDLSCs have also demonstrated potential within regenerative endodontics. Experimental studies show that PDLSCs can differentiate into odontoblast-like cells and participate in dentin formation when introduced into damaged pulp spaces. Their secretory activity also supports angiogenic and immunomodulatory processes within the pulp microenvironment, indicating that PDLSCs can contribute to tissue repair through both direct and paracrine mechanisms. The regenerative capacity of PDLSCs is most clearly illustrated in models of periodontal repair. PDLSCs can generate cementum-like tissue and form organized periodontal ligament fibers that span from the cementum to alveolar bone. This functionality is key to treating periodontal defects arising from chronic inflammatory disease. By contributing to the structural organization and biomechanical resilience of the periodontal ligament, PDLSCs help restore normal tooth support and function. Beyond direct transplantation approaches, PDLSCs have been incorporated into tissue engineering strategies that utilize biodegradable scaffolds to provide 3D support for cell growth and differentiation. These scaffolds mimic ECM architecture and facilitate the formation of organized tissues when combined with PDLSCs. The addition of inductive factors such as BMPs can further enhance differentiation, enabling reconstruction of complex dental and craniofacial structures. Moreover, PDLSCs possess immunomodulatory properties, including the ability to reduce inflammatory cytokine production, which complement their regenerative functions in diseased or infected tissues. Despite their broad potential, several constraints limit the clinical translation of PDLSCs. Obtaining periodontal ligament tissue requires tooth extraction, restricting availability and raising concerns about donor suitability. Cell yield and quality vary with age, systemic health, and periodontal conditions, which introduces variability into downstream applications. As with other dental stem cell types, the lack of standardized procedures for isolation, culture, and therapeutic use remains a significant barrier. Long-term *in vivo* studies and well-designed clinical trials are essential to determine the safety, predictability, and durability of PDLSC-based treatments.

5.2.4 Other dental stem cells

In addition to the widely studied DPSCs and PDLSCs, a number of other stem cell populations derived from dental tissues have gained attention for their regenerative potential. Among these, dental follicle progenitor cells (DFPCs) and gingival mesenchymal stem cells (GMSCs) have emerged as biologically versatile and readily accessible sources for tissue engineering applications. Their unique properties including ease of isolation, multilineage differentiation capacity, and robust paracrine activity broaden the scope of regenerative therapies in dentistry and may extend to craniofacial and systemic applications.

DFPCs originate from the dental follicle, a transient connective tissue that surrounds the developing tooth germ and contributes to tooth eruption. DFPCs are generally collected from unerupted or impacted third molars during extraction procedures. These cells display hallmark mesenchymal features, including strong proliferative capacity and the ability to differentiate into osteoblasts, cementoblasts, and fibroblasts. Their secretory profile, which includes factors such as VEGF and TGF-β, supports angiogenesis and early tissue repair. Preclinical studies indicate that DFPCs can generate cementum-like structures and organized periodontal ligament fibers, underscoring their suitability for periodontal regeneration and other applications requiring reconstruction of mineralized tissues (Volponi et al., 2018). Their utility in alveolar and craniofacial bone regeneration is also being explored, particularly in combination with advanced scaffold systems that promote controlled cell organization and matrix deposition.

GMSCs represent another promising dental-derived stem cell population. GMSCs are isolated from the connective tissue of the gingiva, making them one of the most accessible sources of mesenchymal stem cells in the oral cavity. Their collection does not require tooth extraction, which reduces patient morbidity and facilitates repeated sampling if needed. GMSCs exhibit potent immunomodulatory properties, including the ability to suppress inflammatory responses via secretion of hepatocyte growth factor, interleukin-10, and other regulatory molecules. In addition to their immunoregulatory activity, GMSCs possess multilineage differentiation potential, forming osteoblasts, chondrocytes, and adipocytes under defined conditions. These characteristics support their use in soft-tissue repair, bone regeneration, and broader craniofacial reconstruction efforts.

Studies increasingly point to applications of DFPCs and GMSCs beyond traditional dental tissues. DFPCs have been evaluated for their capacity to enhance alveolar bone formation, particularly when paired with biomaterials engineered to mimic the ECM architecture. GMSCs, owing to their strong immunomodulatory effects, are being studied in models of systemic inflammatory and autoimmune disorders, where they have been shown to reduce inflammatory activity and promote tissue repair. Their ability to support angiogenesis further broadens their potential in regenerative medicine.

Both cell types demonstrate strong compatibility with modern biomaterial platforms. DFPCs seeded onto bioengineered scaffolds have shown success in regenerating periodontal structures, while GMSCs incorporated into hydrogels or polymeric scaffolds display organized growth and enhanced regenerative outcomes in gingival and soft-tissue models. These scaffold-based strategies underscore the importance of integrating cell biology with material engineering to optimize regenerative outcomes. Despite considerable promise, the translation of DFPC- and GMSC-based therapies to clinical practice presents ongoing challenges. Variability in donor tissue, differences in cell yield, and the absence of standardized protocols for isolation and expansion contribute to inconsistencies across studies. Long-term assessment of safety, particularly in relation to potential tumorigenicity or aberrant immune responses, remains essential. Addressing these issues will be critical for advancing DFPCs and GMSCs from experimental systems to clinically reliable components of regenerative dentistry.

5.3 MECHANISMS OF STEM CELL-MEDIATED REGENERATION

Stem cell-mediated regeneration within dental tissues involves a coordinated sequence of cellular events and molecular signaling pathways that collectively drive the restoration of the pulp–dentin complex and associated root structures. These processes depend on the ability of stem cells

Artificial Insect-Inspired Vision for Autonomous Systems

RIVER PUBLISHERS SERIES IN COMMUNICATIONS AND NETWORKING

Series Editors:

ABBAS JAMALIPOUR
The University of Sydney, Australia

MARINA RUGGIERI
University of Rome Tor Vergata, Italy

The "River Publishers Series in Communications and Networking" is a series of comprehensive academic and professional books which focus on communication and network systems. Topics range from the theory and use of systems involving all terminals, computers, and information processors to wired and wireless networks and network layouts, protocols, architectures, and implementations. Also covered are developments stemming from new market demands in systems, products, and technologies such as personal communications services, multimedia systems, enterprise networks, and optical communications.

The series includes research monographs, edited volumes, handbooks and textbooks, providing professionals, researchers, educators, and advanced students in the field with an invaluable insight into the latest research and developments.

Topics included in this series include:-

- Communication theory
- Multimedia systems
- Network architecture
- Optical communications
- Personal communication services
- Telecoms networks
- Wifi network protocols

For a list of other books in this series, visit www.riverpublishers.com

regulators such as Runx2 and Osterix and drive the expression of odontogenic markers including dentin sialophosphoprotein and dentin matrix protein 1. Beyond their effects on lineage commitment, BMPs contribute to the mineralization of newly deposited dentin matrix, which is essential for restoring the structural integrity of regenerated tissue. Preclinical studies have shown that combining BMP-2 with DPSCs can markedly enhance pulp–dentin regeneration, supporting its therapeutic utility in endodontic applications (Hargreaves et al., 2008).

TGF-β, another key mediator of dental tissue repair, performs broader regulatory functions across multiple stages of regeneration. Stored abundantly within the dentin matrix, TGF-β is released following tissue injury and serves as an endogenous signal for initiating repair. Through activation of the Smad signaling pathway, TGF-β modulates genes involved in odontoblast differentiation, ECM synthesis, and cellular recruitment. A notable aspect of TGF-β activity is its ability to promote the homing and mobilization of endogenous stem cells toward the site of injury, thereby facilitating intrinsic repair mechanisms. Its role in ECM organization further contributes to the stability and functional maturation of regenerated pulp–dentin tissue.

Also, VEGF plays a distinct and essential role in establishing a functional vascular network within the regenerating pulp. Angiogenesis is a prerequisite for supporting metabolically active tissues, and VEGF acts by stimulating endothelial cell proliferation, migration, and tubule formation. VEGF also interacts synergistically with BMP and TGF-β pathways, creating a regenerative milieu that encourages both odontogenic differentiation and vascular development. In experimental models of pulp regeneration, VEGF has been shown to promote the formation of vascularized pulp-like tissue, supporting the survival and integration of newly differentiated odontoblast-like cells (Hargreaves et al., 2008). Effective regeneration of the pulp–dentin complex requires the integrated activity of these growth factors. BMPs and TGF-β drive odontoblastic differentiation and matrix deposition, while VEGF ensures the establishment of a vascular supply that sustains the metabolic and functional needs of the regenerating tissue (Figure 5.2). The combined actions of these signaling molecules form a coordinated biological program that restores both the structure and the physiological function of damaged dental tissues.

In regenerative endodontic procedures, these growth factors are frequently incorporated into biomaterial scaffolds to improve their delivery, stability, and bioactivity. Scaffolds emulate the ECM, providing a 3D framework that supports cell attachment, proliferation, and differentiation while enabling the controlled release of growth factors at the site of injury. Preconditioning stem cells with individual or combined growth factors prior to transplantation has also been shown to enhance their regenerative performance, reflecting the importance of synchronizing cell-based therapies with molecular cues.

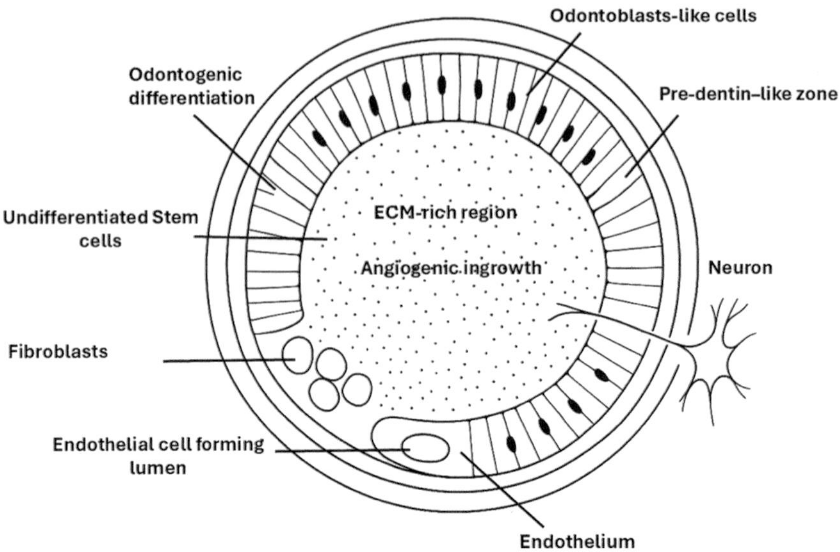

Figure 5.2 Molecular mechanisms that regulate odontoblastic differentiation, vascular formation, and neural ingrowth in regenerative endodontics. The diagram illustrates how BMPs, TGF-β, VEGF, and neurotrophic mediators coordinate stem cell differentiation, angiogenesis, and innervation during pulp–dentin complex regeneration.

Despite their therapeutic promise, several challenges impede the clinical translation of growth factor-mediated regeneration. Achieving precise control over dosage, release kinetics, and local concentration is essential to prevent adverse outcomes such as excessive mineralization or dysregulated tissue growth. Moreover, the complex interactions among different signaling pathways require further elucidation to optimize synergistic effects and minimize unintended responses. Ongoing advances in biomimetic delivery systems, controlled-release technologies, and rational combinations of growth factors are expected to improve the reliability and safety of these approaches and expand their clinical applicability in regenerative dentistry.

5.7 IMPORTANCE OF STEM CELL PLASTICITY IN ACHIEVING FUNCTIONAL REGENERATION

Stem cell plasticity, which is defined as the capacity of stem cells to adopt multiple lineage fates in response to environmental and molecular cues, is fundamental to effective regeneration of dental tissues. This adaptive potential enables dental-derived stem cells to respond dynamically to injury and developmental signals, thereby supporting the restoration of the structural and functional components of the pulp–dentin complex. Recent studies, including those by Krivanek et al. (2023), underscore the fluidity with which dental stem cells transition between different cellular states, highlighting plasticity as a key biological property underpinning their regenerative capability.

The relevance of stem cell plasticity becomes evident in the diverse roles dental stem cells assume during tissue repair. DPSCs, for example, can differentiate into odontoblast-like cells to regenerate dentin, while also contributing to angiogenesis and neurogenesis within the pulp space. This multifunctional capacity supports the re-establishment of essential physiological functions such as nutrient delivery, immune regulation, and sensory activity. Likewise, SCAP display high plasticity, enabling the formation of dentin and facilitating continued root development in immature teeth. These adaptive responses form the basis of regenerative endodontic procedures designed to restore vitality to previously necrotic teeth. Stem cell plasticity is tightly regulated by the stem cell niche, which is a specialized microenvironment that maintains stem cell homeostasis and directs their fate. In continuously growing teeth such as rodent incisors, the niche orchestrates the balance between self-renewal and differentiation, ensuring a constant supply of progenitor cells for tissue maintenance and repair. Krivanek et al. (2023) demonstrated that dental stem cells routinely cycle between quiescent, proliferative, and differentiating states, enabling them to respond efficiently to physiological demands and tissue injury. At the molecular level, plasticity is governed by a network of signaling pathways and extracellular cues. Pathways involving Wnt, BMP, and TGF-β play central roles in regulating gene expression programs associated with self-renewal, lineage specification, and differentiation. The ECM further contributes to this regulation by providing structural anchorage and biochemical stimuli. ECM components such as fibronectin and collagen activate integrin-mediated signaling, which modulates cytoskeletal dynamics and transcriptional responses that influence stem cell behavior. Understanding these regulatory mechanisms has important implications for regenerative endodontics. By identifying key molecular signals that maintain or enhance plasticity, targeted therapies can be developed to direct stem cell differentiation toward specific lineages, such as odontoblast-like cells, endothelial cells, or neural cells. Such strategies could improve the fidelity and functionality of regenerated pulp–dentin tissues. Approaches that combine precise modulation of signaling pathways with advanced biomaterials that replicate the native niche environment show particular promise. However, clinical translation of stem cell plasticity remains challenging. High plasticity carries the risk of unintended or aberrant differentiation, which may compromise tissue functionality. The absence of standard *in vivo* protocols for controlling stem cell state transitions further complicates therapeutic applications. Addressing these limitations will require deeper mechanistic insights into stem cell regulation and the development of biomaterials and delivery systems capable of recreating the native niche with sufficient precision to guide predictable regenerative outcomes.

5.8 INTEGRATION WITH 3D ORGANOID TECHNOLOGY

3D organoid technology has introduced a transformative approach to tissue engineering and regenerative medicine by enabling the development of highly organized *in vitro* models that more accurately reflect native tissue biology. Organoids are self-organized, stem cell-derived constructs that recapitulate key architectural and functional features of their tissue of origin (Table 5.2). In dental research, 3D organoid systems have rapidly gained prominence as valuable platforms for studying pulp and root tissue development, modeling disease processes, and evaluating emerging regenerative strategies. Organoid formation builds on the intrinsic self-organization capacity of stem cells. When cultured under defined conditions, these cells undergo coordinated differentiation and spatial arrangement to form structures that mimic *in vivo* tissue organization. Dental-derived stem cells such as DPSCs and SCAP are particularly well suited for organoid generation because of their strong proliferative capacity and multilineage differentiation tendencies. The resulting dental organoids reproduce characteristic features of pulp and root tissues, including diverse cell populations, ECM deposition, and preliminary tissue patterning, making them highly informative for investigating pulp–dentin complex regeneration. One of the major strengths of 3D organoids lies in their ability to model the microenvironmental interactions that govern tissue development and repair. Dental organoids allow the study of interactions among odontoblast-like cells, endothelial cells, neuronal elements, and ECM components within a single system. This level of biological complexity is not achievable with conventional two-dimensional cultures. Organoids, therefore, serve as dynamic models for examining dentinogenesis, angiogenesis, and neurogenesis. In studies of pulp regeneration, organoid systems have proven particularly useful for examining the processes underlying the formation of vascularized and innervated pulp-like tissues. When dental stem cells are cultured with defined angiogenic and neurogenic signals, the resulting organoids develop microvascular networks and neural structures that resemble those found in native pulp. These models provide a controlled environment for investigating the molecular pathways that drive vascular and neural integration, both of which are essential for restoring the vitality and function of regenerated pulp tissue (Figure 5.3).

Organoid models have also been applied to the study of root development. Using SCAP, researchers have generated organoids that replicate early stages of root formation, including odontoblast differentiation and

Table 5.2 3D organoid models in dental tissue regeneration

Organoid type	*Cell source*	*Features*	*Applications*
Pulp–dentin organoids	DPSCs and SCAP	Vascularized, dentin-producing cells	Pulp–dentin complex regeneration
Periodontal organoids	PDLSCs	Cementum and ligament-like structures	Periodontal tissue repair
Root development organoids	SCAP	Root elongation and dentinogenesis	Modeling root maturation and apexogenesis
Neuralized dental organoids	DPSCs, NGF-treated cells	Nerve-like networks within pulp	Restoring pulp innervation and sensory functions

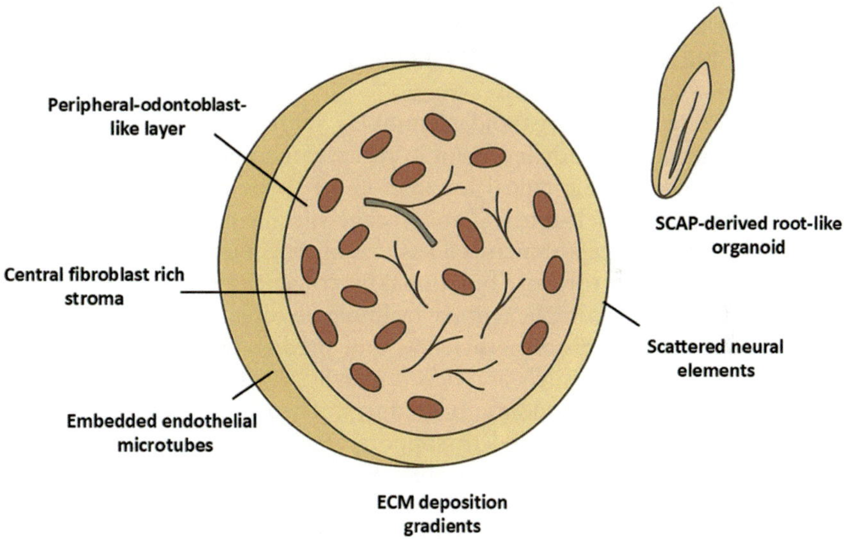

Figure 5.3 Structural organization of dental organoids generated from dental-derived stem cells. The schematic shows spatial arrangement of odontoblast-like cells, fibroblasts, endothelial networks, neural elements, and extracellular matrix within 3D organoid constructs that model pulp and root tissue development.

dentin matrix deposition. These systems offer valuable insights into the mechanisms of root elongation and maturation and provide an experimental platform for testing regenerative approaches aimed at managing immature teeth with incomplete root development. The integration of organoid technology with regenerative endodontics holds considerable promise for advancing therapeutic applications. By combining organoids with engineered biomaterials such as hydrogels or nanofibrous scaffolds, it is possible to create hybrid constructs that mimic the structural and functional features of the native pulp–dentin complex. Early studies suggest that such constructs may be suitable for transplantation into root canals to promote functional tissue regeneration, offering a potential alternative to conventional endodontic procedures. Despite these advances, several challenges must be addressed before organoid-based approaches can be translated to clinical practice. Standardized methodologies for organoid generation including stem cell selection, culture matrices, and differentiation protocols are needed to improve reproducibility across laboratories. Scaling organoid production for therapeutic use remains an additional obstacle. Furthermore, achieving stable integration of organoids with host tissues and ensuring their long-term function and safety *in vivo* are critical questions that require further investigation.

5.9 SYNERGY BETWEEN ORGANOIDS AND STEM CELL-BASED APPROACHES IN REGENERATIVE ENDODONTICS

The integration of 3D organoid technology with stem cell-based strategies represents a major advancement in regenerative endodontics. Stem cell therapies provide the biological foundation for tissue repair through their inherent capacity for self-renewal and lineage-specific differentiation, while organoid systems offer a structured *in vitro* microenvironment that closely replicates the architecture and functional heterogeneity of native dental tissues. Together, these complementary technologies create a robust platform that enhances the precision, efficiency, and predictability of regenerative approaches. Stem cells such as DPSCs and SCAP have long formed the basis of regenerative endodontic procedures. Their ability to differentiate into odontoblast-like cells and to support vascular and neural regeneration underpins their therapeutic utility. However, optimal differentiation and functional integration require a physiological microenvironment and reliable exposure to inductive signals. Organoid technology addresses this need by recreating key aspects of the native stem cell niche, enabling more accurate control over cell behavior, lineage specification, and maturation. The strength of this combined approach lies in its ability to overcome limitations inherent to each technique. Traditional stem cell-based systems often struggle to recapitulate the complex spatial organization and cell–cell interactions characteristic of dental tissues. Organoids, by contrast, self-organize into stratified, heterogeneous structures that reflect the cellular and extracellular organization of the pulp–dentin complex. When stem cells are incorporated into organoid cultures, they benefit from an environment that promotes survival, proliferation, and directed differentiation. This integration results in constructs that more closely approximate the biological features of native pulp and root tissues and enhances the overall regenerative outcome. One of the most compelling applications of this synergy is in the generation of bioengineered pulp tissue. By combining stem cells with 3D dental organoids, researchers have created vascularized and innervated pulp-like constructs that reproduce essential physiological functions, including nutrient exchange, sensory signaling, and immune defense. These engineered tissues can potentially be transplanted into root canals to support complete revitalization of teeth, offering a biologically based alternative to conventional root canal therapy and extending the lifespan of compromised teeth. The combined approach also has significant implications for root regeneration. Organoids derived from SCAP can mimic early root development, including odontoblast differentiation and dentin matrix deposition. When used alongside stem cell therapies, these organoids provide controlled systems for examining the mechanisms of root maturation and for evaluating new regeneration strategies. This is particularly relevant for the management of immature teeth with necrotic pulp, where current treatments fail to promote adequate root development or strengthen the root structure. Beyond direct therapeutic applications, the integration of organoids with stem cell-based approaches accelerates mechanistic research in regenerative endodontics. Organoids allow detailed examination of the interactions among stem cells, signaling molecules, and biomaterials in a 3D context. They can be used to investigate the effects of growth factors such as BMPs, TGF-β, and VEGF on cell behavior and to assess the biocompatibility and performance of scaffolds and delivery systems. These insights contribute to the refinement of regenerative protocols and facilitate the translation of laboratory findings to clinical practice.

5.10 CASE STUDIES ON INTEGRATING ORGANOIDS AND STEM CELLS IN DENTAL REGENERATION

The introduction of organoid technologies into regenerative medicine was profoundly shaped by the work of Lancaster and Knoblich (2014), who demonstrated that stem cell-derived structures possess an intrinsic capacity for self-organization into tissue-like architectures. Their studies showed that organoids can reproduce key aspects of the native tissue morphology and function *in vitro*, thereby providing highly controlled platforms for examining development, disease, and repair. This conceptual breakthrough established organoids as powerful tools for modeling tissue complexity, offering new opportunities for investigating cellular behavior, lineage specification, and microenvironmental interactions. The principles defined in their work laid the groundwork for utilizing organoids in dental tissue engineering, where recreating the architectural and functional characteristics of the pulp–dentin complex is essential for meaningful regeneration.

Building on this foundational framework, Krivanek et al. (2023) applied organoid systems directly to the study of dental tissues. Their work demonstrated that organoids generated from dental-derived stem cells can mimic critical aspects of pulp and root biology, including dentinogenesis, vascularization, and early root development. By incorporating DPSCs and SCAP into 3D culture environments, the researchers were able to recreate tissue-specific microenvironments and analyze cell behavior under conditions that closely resemble *in vivo* development. Their findings emphasize the importance of organoid–stem cell integration for modeling disease, studying repair mechanisms, and designing regenerative strategies capable of supporting root maturation in immature teeth. Advances in organoid customization and engineering described by Takebe and Wells (2019) further expanded the therapeutic potential of these systems. Their work highlighted innovations in genetic manipulation, biomaterial integration, and microengineering that enhance the precision, reproducibility, and functional relevance of organoids. Such technological refinements enable organoids to serve as highly tunable platforms for regenerative dental research. When combined with stem cell-based approaches, engineered organoids can simulate the niche environment required for guiding stem cell differentiation, improving tissue organization, and promoting integration of regenerated structures. These capabilities are directly relevant to dental tissue engineering, where precise control over cell fate and tissue architecture is crucial for restoring the pulp–dentin complex.

The regenerative capacity of dental stem/progenitor cells was demonstrated convincingly by Huang et al. (2010), who showed that DPSCs combined with appropriate scaffolding materials can regenerate vascularized and innervated pulp-like tissue while concurrently forming continuous layers of dentin. These findings provided a practical foundation for integrating stem cells with organoid platforms to achieve functional regeneration. By coupling the structural and environmental advantages of organoids with the multilineage potency of dental stem cells, researchers can address both the architectural and physiological requirements of dental tissue repair. Collectively, these studies highlight the strong synergy that emerges when organoid technology is combined with stem cell-based regenerative approaches. Organoids offer the architectural framework and microenvironmental signals that are needed to model complex tissue interactions, while stem cells supply the regenerative and differentiation capacities necessary for functional restoration. This integrated strategy enhances the mechanistic understanding of dental tissue development and provides a pathway toward therapeutic innovations that move beyond conventional endodontic treatments. As organoid engineering and stem cell biology continue to evolve, their combined application holds significant promise for achieving comprehensive, biologically driven regeneration of damaged dental tissues.

5.11 SCAFFOLDS AND BIOMATERIALS IN REGENERATIVE ENDODONTICS

Scaffolds are a central component of regenerative endodontics because they provide the structural support and biological context required for stem cell-mediated tissue repair. Their primary function is to recreate features of the natural ECM, allowing stem cells to attach, survive, and differentiate within the root canal space (Figure 5.4). By offering both mechanical stability and biochemical signals, scaffolds help guide the organized formation of new pulp and dentin tissues. A key role of scaffolds is to maintain stem cells within the site of regeneration. The 3D frameworks prevent cell loss and allow cells to distribute evenly throughout the construct, which is essential for producing uniform and functional tissue. By mimicking the physical properties of the native ECM, scaffolds support cell migration and encourage the formation of continuous layers of odontoblast-like cells along the dentinal walls.

Scaffolds also contribute to regeneration by delivering biochemical signals that influence cell fate. These signals may derive from the scaffold material itself or from incorporated molecules such as BMPs, TGF-β, or VEGF. Odontogenic factors promote differentiation toward an odontoblastic phenotype, leading to deposition of dentin matrix, while angiogenic factors support the formation of a vascular network within the regenerating pulp tissue. Incorporating such molecules into scaffold systems allows controlled, localized presentation of signals that enhance tissue specificity and regenerative efficacy. Spatial organization is another important function of scaffolds. By providing defined boundaries and structural

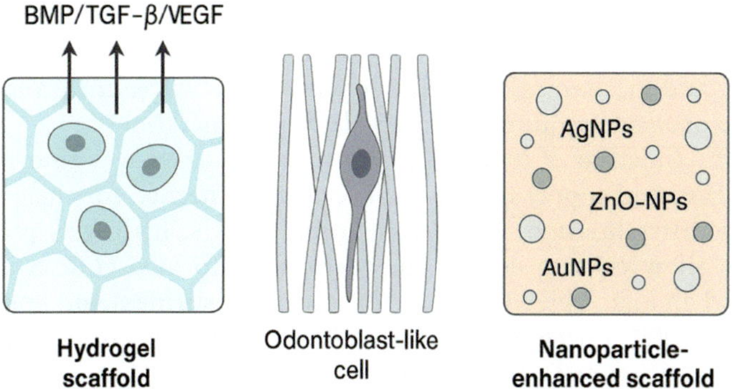

Figure 5.4 Biomaterial scaffolds that are used in regenerative endodontics. The figure compares hydrogel systems, nanofibrous scaffolds, and nanoparticle-enhanced constructs, illustrating their structural characteristics and roles in supporting stem cell retention, differentiation, vascularization, and antimicrobial activity.

orientation, scaffolds help regulate the growth pattern of regenerating pulp tissue and prevent disorganized or excessive cell proliferation. Hydrogels are frequently used for this purpose because of their biocompatibility and ability to encapsulate cells and growth factors in a hydrated environment similar to native pulp. Nanofibrous scaffolds, which reproduce the fibrous architecture of the ECM, support cell alignment and offer greater mechanical strength, making them suitable for reconstructing more complex pulp–dentin interfaces. In addition to supporting stem cells, scaffolds can serve as delivery systems for therapeutic agents. Incorporating antimicrobial or anti-inflammatory compounds helps address infection and inflammation, which are common barriers to successful regeneration. This multifunctional capacity makes scaffolds a versatile element of regenerative endodontic treatment strategies.

Several challenges still limit the widespread clinical use of scaffolds. Ensuring biocompatibility and appropriate degradation rates is essential as materials must support tissue formation without causing inflammation or interfering with healing. Mechanical properties must be tuned to withstand forces within the root canal while remaining conducive to cell infiltration and matrix deposition. Further advances in material design are needed to more accurately reproduce the complex biochemical and mechanical characteristics of the native ECM and to improve integration with host tissues.

5.12 BIOMATERIAL DESIGN FOR ENDODONTIC APPLICATIONS: HYDROGEL SYSTEMS FOR PULP–DENTIN COMPLEX REGENERATION

Hydrogels play an important role in regenerative endodontics because they provide a 3D environment that supports stem cell survival and organization while resembling key features of the native ECM. Their hydrated structure, porosity, and mechanical tunability make them suitable for promoting the sequence of events required for pulp–dentin regeneration.

A major function of hydrogels is to maintain DPSCs within the site of regeneration and supply the physical conditions needed for their proliferation and differentiation. By encapsulating DPSCs, hydrogels prevent cell loss and allow cells to occupy the scaffold uniformly. Han et al. (2024) developed an injectable hydrogel with controlled stiffness and porosity that supported DPSC differentiation into odontogenic and endothelial lineages. The system produced vascularized pulp-like tissue and continuous dentin deposition, showing that hydrogel properties directly influence lineage outcomes during regeneration. Hydrogels also act as carriers for bioactive molecules that regulate stem cell behavior. Growth factors such as BMPs, TGF-β, and VEGF are frequently incorporated to guide odontoblast differentiation and vascularization. Zhang et al. (2024) reported a GelMA-based hydrogel containing carbon dot nanozymes, which reduced oxidative stress in inflamed pulp tissue and improved dentin formation. The ability to release bioactive signals in a controlled manner is one of the main reasons hydrogels are widely used in pulp–dentin tissue engineering.

Hydrogels can also incorporate therapeutic agents that address inflammation or infection. These two factors often interfere with regeneration. Ma and Xu (2024) developed a nanocomposite hydrogel combining curcumin-loaded chitosan nanoparticles with DPSC-conditioned media. The system showed anti-inflammatory and antioxidative activity and improved pulp healing and dentinogenesis in preclinical work. These results demonstrate that hydrogels can simultaneously manage the injury environment and support tissue repair. Injectable hydrogels are particularly useful in endodontics because they adapt to the narrow and irregular anatomy of the root canal system. Materials such as alginate, GelMA, and PEG form gels *in situ*, filling the canal space and providing mechanical support while remaining permeable to nutrients. Their physical properties can be adjusted to match conditions that allow stem cells to survive and deposit new matrix.

Hydrogels are also used to co-culture DPSCs with endothelial or neural progenitor cells to promote vascular and neural development in regenerated tissue. Dissanayaka et al. (2023) demonstrated that hydrogels containing DPSCs and endothelial cells formed organized vascular networks, an essential requirement for sustaining regenerated pulp tissue.

5.13 NANOPARTICLE-ENHANCED SCAFFOLDS FOR ANTIMICROBIAL AND REGENERATIVE PROPERTIES

Nanoparticle-enhanced scaffolds have emerged as an important development in regenerative endodontics because they address two major requirements of the root canal environment, controlling infection and supporting tissue regeneration. Incorporation of nanoparticles such as silver (AgNPs), zinc oxide (ZnO-NPs), and gold (AuNPs) into scaffold matrices provides antimicrobial and pro-regenerative properties within a single system (Table 5.3). This combined functionality is particularly relevant in endodontics, where persistent infection and inadequate tissue repair are primary reasons for treatment failure. The antimicrobial activity of nanoparticle-modified scaffolds is one of their most effective attributes. AgNPs demonstrate broad-spectrum activity against common endodontic pathogens, including *Streptococcus mutans* and *Enterococcus faecalis*. Niska et al. (2016) reported that scaffolds loaded with AgNPs exert sustained antimicrobial effects through the controlled release of silver ions. This continuous activity helps maintain a sterile environment, reducing the likelihood of reinfection while creating conditions suitable for tissue

Table 5.3 Nanoparticle-enhanced scaffolds for dental regeneration

Nanoparticles	*Function*	*Advantage*
Silver (AgNPs)	Antimicrobial	Reduces bacterial colonization in root canals
Zinc oxide (ZnO-NPs)	Promotes odontogenic differentiation	Enhances dentin mineralization
Gold (AuNPs)	Growth factor delivery	Improves osteogenic and dentinogenic potential
Hydroxyapatite (HA-NPs)	Biomineralization	Supports dentin and enamel repair

repair. AgNPs disrupt microbial membranes, alter metabolic pathways, and interfere with DNA replication, making them effective in environments where conventional disinfectants have limited penetration. Nanoparticles also contribute directly to regenerative processes. ZnO-NPs, for example, enhance the odontogenic differentiation of DPSCs. When incorporated into scaffold structures, ZnO-NPs promote mineralized matrix formation and support dentin regeneration, aiding the repair of the pulp–dentin complex. Several systems have been developed to integrate regenerative signals into nanoparticle-enhanced scaffolds. AuNPs are frequently used because of their biocompatibility and ability to bind bioactive molecules. Niska et al. (2016) demonstrated that scaffolds functionalized with AuNPs and growth factors such as BMPs accelerated mineralized tissue formation and improved overall regenerative outcomes. These multifunctional scaffolds combine structural support with targeted delivery of signaling molecules, increasing their utility in endodontic applications.

Nanoparticle incorporation also influences the mechanical and physicochemical properties of scaffolds. Polymers such as polylactic acid and chitosan are commonly used as base materials because they are biodegradable and compatible with nanoparticle integration. Adjusting nanoparticle concentration, size, and release kinetics allows tuning of scaffold performance, balancing antimicrobial activity with cytocompatibility and mechanical stability within the root canal environment. Despite the promising results, several issues need to be addressed before nanoparticle-enhanced scaffolds can be used clinically. Ensuring biocompatibility and minimizing cytotoxicity remain essential as the biological effects of nanoparticles can vary with the dose and release rate. Long-term stability, interaction with host tissues, and functional behavior under *in vivo* conditions, including moisture, enzymatic degradation, and mechanical loading, require further investigation. Continued refinement of nanoparticle formulations and scaffold architectures will be necessary to translate these systems into predictable clinical tools.

5.14 CHALLENGES AND FUTURE DIRECTIONS

Stem cell-based regenerative endodontics offers substantial potential for restoring damaged dental tissues, yet several challenges must be addressed before these therapies can be widely implemented. Among these, immune compatibility and ethical considerations remain central concerns, influencing both clinical safety and regulatory acceptance.

Immune compatibility is a major barrier when introducing exogenous cells into the pulp–dentin complex. Allogeneic stem cells, although attractive due to their availability and scalability, may trigger host immune responses that lead to rejection or diminished therapeutic activity. Approaches to mitigate these responses include reducing stem cell immunogenicity through genetic modification, administering immunosuppressive agents, or using encapsulation systems that provide physical protection from immune surveillance. The development of induced pluripotent stem cells (iPSCs) has added an alternative route as iPSCs can be derived from the patient and expanded into autologous cell populations with minimal immunological risk. However, personalized iPSC-based therapies are hindered by high production costs, extended processing times, and complex quality control requirements.

Ethical considerations also influence the development and acceptance of stem cell-based endodontic therapies. The use of embryonic stem cells (ESCs) remains ethically sensitive due to concerns surrounding embryo destruction during cell derivation. Although ESCs possess strong regenerative potential, these ethical constraints have shifted focus toward adult stem cell sources such as DPSCs and SCAP, which are more accessible and largely free of ethical controversy. iPSCs also avoid embryo-related concerns, further supporting their suitability for translational applications.

The commercialization of stem cell therapies raises additional ethical issues related to cost, accessibility, and equity. The high expense associated with generating, expanding, and delivering stem cell products may limit availability to patients with greater socioeconomic resources. Ensuring equitable access will require coordinated strategies involving regulatory bodies, clinicians, and industry partners to balance innovation with affordability.

Long-term safety is another critical consideration. While preclinical and early clinical studies demonstrate promising outcomes, the risks of tumorigenesis, inappropriate differentiation, or ectopic tissue formation remain. These risks emphasize the need for robust regulatory frameworks capable of evaluating stem cell-based products, monitoring clinical outcomes, and enforcing long-term follow-up. Transparent reporting of both therapeutic successes and adverse events will be essential to maintain clinician and patient confidence.

Despite these challenges, progress continues through advances in biomaterials, gene editing, and cell engineering. Immunomodulatory scaffolds, nanoparticle-based delivery systems, and CRISPR-/Cas9-mediated gene editing offer potential solutions for reducing immunogenicity and improving regenerative efficacy. Ongoing research is also focused on optimizing culture protocols, refining delivery approaches, and developing scalable manufacturing systems to reduce costs and improve consistency.

5.15 SUMMARY

This chapter summarized the principles and current progress of stem cell-based regenerative endodontics. It outlined the limitations of conventional root canal therapy and presented regenerative endodontics as an approach aimed at restoring biological function within the pulp–dentin complex. The discussion highlighted the contributions of DPSCs, SCAP, and PDLSCs, emphasizing their proliferation, differentiation, and paracrine activity in supporting pulp regeneration, dentin formation, and root maturation. Advances in biomaterials were reviewed, including hydrogels, scaffolds, and nanoparticle-modified systems that provide structural support, guide cell behavior, and assist in controlling microbial and inflammatory challenges. The application of 3D organoid models was also examined, besides discussing the key regenerative mechanisms, including odontoblastic differentiation, angiogenesis, and neurogenesis with reference to the growth factors and signaling pathways that regulate them. Important gaps remain, particularly in managing immune responses, addressing ethical constraints, and establishing uniform clinical protocols. These issues continue to limit consistent translation into practice. Even so, current findings support the feasibility of stem cell-mediated regeneration as a future direction in endodontic therapy. Further refinement of stem cell sources, biomaterial systems, and controlled *in vivo* studies will be required to develop approaches that are reliable and clinically reproducible.

REFERENCES

Dissanayaka, W. L., Zhang, Z., & Nör, J. E. (2023). Stem cell and endothelial cell co-culture systems for vascularized dental pulp regeneration. *Frontiers in Dental Medicine*, 4, 1094927.

Gronthos, S., Mankani, M., Brahim, J., Robey, P. G., & Shi, S. (2000). Postnatal human dental pulp stem cells (DPSCs) in vitro and in vivo. *Proceedings of the National Academy of Sciences*, 97(25), 13625–13630.

Han, Y., Xu, J., Chopra, H., Zhang, Z., Dubey, N., Dissanayaka, W. L., Nör, J. E., & Bottino, M. C. (2024). Injectable tissue-specific hydrogel system for pulp–dentin regeneration. *Journal of Dental Research*, 103(4), 398–408.

Hargreaves, K. M., Giesler, T., Henry, M., & Wang, Y. (2008). Regeneration potential of the young permanent tooth: What does the future hold? *Journal of Endodontics*, 34(7), S51–S56.

Huang, G. T., Yamaza, T., Shea, L. D., Djouad, F., Kuhn, N. Z., Tuan, R. S., & Shi, S. (2010). Stem/progenitor cell-mediated de novo regeneration of dental pulp with newly deposited continuous layers of dentin in an in vivo model. *Tissue Engineering Part A*, 16(2), 605–615.

Huang, X., Huang, G. T., & Shi, S. (2020). Mesenchymal stem cells derived from dental tissues: Regenerative potential, therapeutic applications, and challenges. *Journal of Endodontics*, 46(4), 509–517.

Krivanek, J., Buchtova, M., Fried, K., & Adameyko, I. (2023). Plasticity of dental cell types in development, regeneration, and evolution. *Journal of Dental Research*, 102(6), 589–598.

Lancaster, M. A., & Knoblich, J. A. (2014). Organogenesis in a dish: Modeling development and disease using organoid technologies. *Science*, 345(6194), 1247125.

Ma, B., & Xu, R. (2024). Dental pulp regeneration via dental pulp stem cells conditioned media and curcumin-loaded nanocomposite hydrogel: An in vitro and in vivo study. *Materials Science-Poland*, 42(2), 113–124.

Niska, K., Knapczyk-Korczak, J., Kowalska, J., & Wysokowski, M. (2016). Antimicrobial and regenerative properties of silver nanoparticle-enriched scaffolds for tissue engineering applications. *International Journal of Nanomedicine*, 11, 2773–2790.

Seo, B. M., Miura, M., Gronthos, S., Bartold, P. M., Batouli, S., Brahim, J., Young, M., Robey, P. G., Wang, C.-Y., & Shi, S. (2004). Investigation of multipotent postnatal stem cells from human periodontal ligament. *The Lancet*, 364(9429), 149–155.

Takebe, T., & Wells, J. M. (2019). Organoids by design. *Science*, 364(6444), 956–959.

Volponi, A. A., Zaugg, L. K., Neves, V., & Sharpe, P. T. (2018). Dental stem cells: A promising tool for regenerative therapy. *Frontiers in Physiology*, 9, 664.

Zhang, Y., Huang, X., Luo, Y., Ma, X., Luo, L., Liang, L., Deng, T., Qiao, Y., Ye, F., & Liao, H. (2024). A carbon dot nanozyme hydrogel enhances pulp regeneration activity by regulating oxidative stress in dental pulpitis. *Journal of Nanobiotechnology*, 22(1), 537.

Chapter 6

Extracellular vesicles in regenerative endodontics

6.1 INTRODUCTION

Extracellular vesicles (EVs) have emerged as an important player in regenerative endodontics, which offers a biologically sophisticated, cell-free alternative that bridges the limitations of conventional stem cell-based therapies with the growing demand for scalable, safe, and highly efficient regenerative solutions. By facilitating the transfer of proteins, lipids, and nucleic acids between cells, EVs serve as fundamental regulators of intercellular communication. Through these molecular exchanges, they exert a profound influence on cellular behavior, including differentiation, angiogenesis, immunomodulation, and matrix synthesis, thereby establishing themselves as potent therapeutic agents for dental tissue regeneration. This chapter presents the biology, classification, functional roles, and translational potential of EVs in regenerative endodontics. They are lipid bilayer-enclosed structures secreted by nearly all mammalian cell types and are involved in a wide array of physiological and pathological processes, including inflammation, development, wound healing, and tumor progression (Table 6.1). EVs are broadly categorized according to their biogenesis, physicochemical properties, and modes of release into three principal subtypes: exosomes, microvesicles, and apoptotic bodies (Figure 6.1).

A. Exosomes: Exosomes are nano-sized vesicles typically measuring 30–150 nm in diameter. They arise through the endosomal pathway, wherein intraluminal vesicles form within multivesicular bodies that subsequently fuse with the plasma membrane to release their contents extracellularly. Exosomes are enriched with microRNAs, tetraspanins, heat shock proteins, lipids, and signaling molecules that enable them to modulate gene expression and cellular responses in a highly targeted manner. Their small size and endosomal origin allow them to traverse tissue barriers efficiently, contributing to their prominence as the most extensively investigated EV subtype in regenerative medicine (Théry et al., 2018).

DOI: 10.1201/9781003589921-6

Table 6.1 Extracellular vesicles and their properties

Type of EV	*Size range*	*Biogenesis*	*Key molecular cargo*	*Functional role in regeneration*
Exosomes	30–150 nm	Endosomal pathway (multivesicular bodies)	MicroRNAs, proteins (tetraspanins), and lipids	Odontogenic differentiation and immune modulation
Microvesicles	100–1000 nm	Direct plasma membrane shedding	Cytokines, adhesion molecules, and growth factors	Angiogenesis and immune response modulation
Apoptotic bodies	1–5 µm	Released during apoptosis	DNA fragments and cellular debris	Tissue remodeling and immunogenic signaling

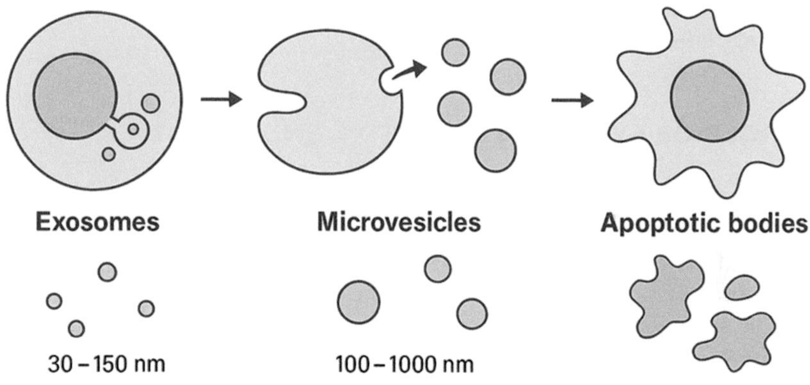

Figure 6.1 Biogenesis and principal subclasses of extracellular vesicles (EVs). Exosomes arise from inward budding of the endosomal membrane and release of intraluminal vesicles from multivesicular bodies. Microvesicles are shed directly from the plasma membrane by outward budding and fission. Apoptotic bodies are larger membrane-bound fragments generated during programmed cell death.

B. Microvesicles: Microvesicles range from approximately 100 to 1000 nm and are generated by outward budding and fission of the plasma membrane. Unlike exosomes, which originate through an intracellular endosomal route, microvesicles are shed directly from the cell surface. They encapsulate molecular cargo reflective of the donor cell's phenotype and functional state, including cytokines, transcription factors, and membrane receptors. Microvesicles are instrumental in processes such as immunoregulation, angiogenesis, and tissue repair, and they contribute significantly to extracellular matrix (ECM) remodeling within injured dental tissues.

C. Apoptotic Bodies: Apoptotic bodies are the largest EV subtype, ranging between 1 and 5 µm in diameter. Released during programmed cell death, they package cellular organelles, chromatin fragments, and cytoplasmic components. Although historically regarded as by-products of apoptosis, apoptotic bodies are increasingly recognized for their potential to modulate immune responses, promote clearance of cellular debris, and influence early phases of tissue repair. Their role in regenerative endodontics, while less explored, represents an emerging area of interest.

The molecular composition of EVs is highly dependent on their cellular source and physiological state. Their cargo includes structural and signaling proteins such as heat shock proteins, integrins, and tetraspanins; bioactive lipids including ceramides and cholesterol; and a wide repertoire of nucleic acids, notably microRNAs and messenger RNAs. Collectively, these molecules equip EVs with the capacity to regulate gene expression, activate intracellular pathways, and modulate the phenotypic behavior of recipient cells.

6.2 ROLE OF EVs IN REGENERATIVE ENDODONTICS

Regenerative endodontics seeks to re-establish the biological architecture and functional integrity of the dental pulp–dentin complex, a goal often compromised by microbial infection, traumatic injury, or developmental disturbances. Conventional approaches such as root canal therapy, although effective at infection control, do not restore the tooth's native vitality or its capacity for sensory function, immune defense, or dentinogenesis. In contrast, EVs offer a biologically active, cell-free strategy capable of orchestrating multiple reparative processes simultaneously, positioning them as a compelling therapeutic alternative in the field (Table 6.2). The promotion of odontogenic differentiation represents one of the most extensively studied regenerative mechanisms mediated by EVs. Vesicles derived from mesenchymal stem cell populations, particularly dental pulp stem cells (DPSCs) and stem cells from the apical papilla (SCAP), are enriched with microRNAs such as miR-21 and miR-218, as well as signaling proteins associated with BMP and Wnt pathways. These molecular constituents activate intracellular programs that drive progenitor cells toward odontoblast-like phenotypes. Experimental evidence demonstrates that such vesicles enhance the deposition of dentin-like matrix *in vitro* and promote mineralized tissue formation *in vivo*, underscoring their potential as biologically guided tools for dentin regeneration (Ivica et al., 2021).

The re-vitalization of the dental pulp also requires the establishment of robust vascular and neural networks. EVs contribute significantly to these

Table 6.2 EV-derived growth factors and their role in regenerative endodontics

Growth factors	*Function*	*Regenerative role in endodontics*
Bone morphogenetic proteins (BMPs)	Induces odontoblast differentiation	Stimulates dentinogenesis and pulp repair
Transforming growth factor-beta (TGF-β)	Regulates cell proliferation and ECM synthesis	Enhances odontoblast differentiation and matrix deposition
Vascular endothelial growth factor (VEGF)	Stimulates blood vessel formation	Improves pulp tissue vascularization
Platelet-derived growth factor (PDGF)	Promotes fibroblast proliferation	Supports periodontal and dentin regeneration
Nerve growth factor (NGF)	Enhances neural differentiation	Promotes pulp innervation and sensory function restoration

processes by transporting pro-angiogenic mediators, including vascular endothelial growth factor (VEGF) and fibroblast growth factor (FGF), which stimulate endothelial proliferation, migration, and tubulogenesis. Simultaneously, the delivery of neurotrophic molecules supports neuronal survival, axonal extension, and integration, thereby enhancing the functional competence of regenerated pulp tissue. These combined angiogenic and neurogenic properties markedly improve the prospects for achieving a vital, fully integrated pulp microenvironment (Kong et al., 2023).

Controlled modulation of the inflammatory response is essential for successful regeneration. EVs have demonstrated notable immunoregulatory capabilities through the delivery of anti-inflammatory cytokines such as IL-10 and regulatory microRNAs including miR-146a. These factors attenuate pro-inflammatory cascades and direct macrophage polarization from the M1 toward the M2 phenotype, fostering a reparative microenvironment conducive to tissue restoration. By mitigating excessive immune activation while promoting constructive remodeling, vesicles help maintain the delicate balance required for predictable healing outcomes (Gholami et al., 2021).

EVs derived specifically from dental stem cells constitute a particularly promising therapeutic platform in regenerative endodontics. These vesicles encapsulate a diverse array of bioactive molecules, including structural proteins, signaling lipids, and regulatory nucleic acids, providing a multifaceted mechanism for influencing cellular behavior and guiding tissue repair (Table 6.3). Their application presents a practical alternative to cell transplantation approaches, circumventing challenges associated with stem cell viability, engraftment, and regulatory complexity.

Dental stem cells comprise a specialized subset of mesenchymal stem cells distinguished by their robust proliferative capacity, multilineage differentiation potential, and relative accessibility from dental tissues. Among these, DPSCs, SCAP, and periodontal ligament stem cells (PLDSCs) are of

Table 6.3 EVs from dental stem cells and their functional roles

EV source	*Key molecular cargo*	*Role in pulp–dentin regeneration*
Dental pulp stem cells (DPSCs)	miR-21, VEGF, BMP-2, and BMP-7	Odontogenic differentiation and angiogenesis
Stem cells from the apical papilla (SCAP)	miR-140–5p, BMP-2, and neurotrophic factors	Root development, apexogenesis, and neurogenesis
Periodontal ligament stem cells (PDLSCs)	VEGF, IL-8, and ECM proteins	PDL regeneration and, immune modulation
Induced pluripotent stem cells (iPSCs)	Customizable EV contents	Personalized regenerative therapies

particular interest due to their developmental proximity to odontogenic and periodontal structures. EVs secreted by these cell populations exhibit a molecular signature uniquely tailored to dental tissue regeneration. They are enriched with odontogenic microRNAs, pro-angiogenic growth factors, and immunomodulatory mediators that collectively promote differentiation toward odontoblast-like phenotypes, support vascular ingrowth, and temper inflammatory responses within the injured microenvironment.

This constellation of bioactive properties positions dental stem cell-derived EVs as highly effective biological agents for restoring the pulp–dentin complex, offering advantages that surpass those of vesicles derived from nondental mesenchymal sources.

DPSCs represent one of the most thoroughly characterized stem cell populations in dental tissue engineering. Isolated from the pulp of permanent teeth, DPSCs display a high proliferative capacity and a robust potential for multilineage differentiation. Critically, they are uniquely predisposed to differentiate into odontoblast-like cells, enabling the formation of reparative dentin and making them central to biologically based approaches for pulp–dentin regeneration.

6.3 DENTAL STEM CELL SOURCES AND THEIR EXTRACELLULAR VESICLE PROFILES

In regenerative endodontics, the therapeutic efficacy of EVs is closely influenced by the biological characteristics of the stem cells from which they originate. Dental tissues harbor several distinct mesenchymal stem cell populations that differ in developmental origin, proliferative behavior, and regenerative specialization. These differences are reflected in the molecular composition of their secreted vesicles, shaping their respective capacities for odontogenic differentiation, angiogenesis, neurogenesis, and immunomodulation. Therefore, characterizing the major dental stem cell sources and understanding the unique regenerative signatures of their EVs are essential for determining their suitability for targeted pulp–dentin repair (Figure 6.2).

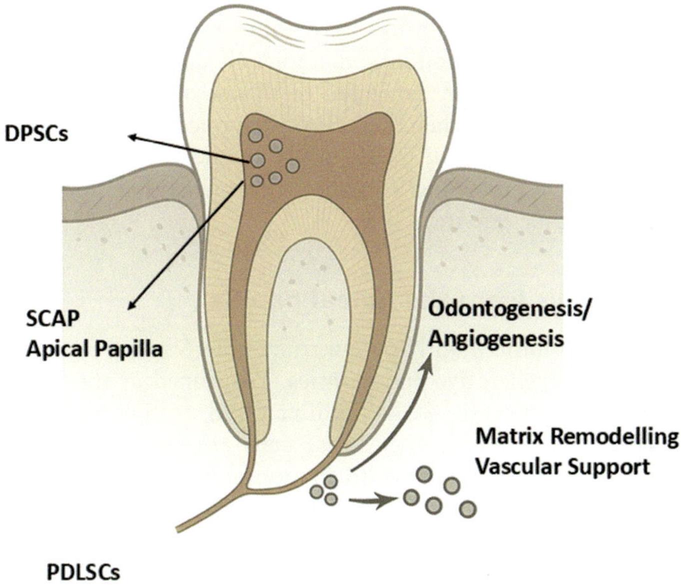

Figure 6.2 Major dental stem cell sources for EVs in regenerative endodontics. Dental pulp stem cells (DPSCs) within the pulp chamber, stem cells from the apical papilla (SCAP) at the root apex, and periodontal ligament stem cells (PDLSCs) along the periodontal ligament secrete EVs with distinct molecular profiles. DPSC-derived vesicles preferentially support odontogenic differentiation and vascular ingrowth, SCAP-derived vesicles contribute to apexogenesis and root maturation, and PDLSC-derived vesicles assist matrix remodeling and microvascular support within the pulp–dentin complex.

6.3.1 Dental pulp stem cells

DPSCs represent one of the most thoroughly characterized stem cell populations in dental tissue engineering. Isolated from the pulp of permanent teeth, DPSCs display a high proliferative capacity and a robust potential for multilineage differentiation. Critically, they are uniquely predisposed to differentiate into odontoblast-like cells, enabling the formation of reparative dentin and making them central to biologically based approaches for pulp–dentin regeneration. EVs derived from DPSCs contain a diverse repertoire of bioactive molecules that directly support regenerative processes. These vesicles are enriched with pro-angiogenic growth factors such as VEGF, as well as members of the bone morphogenetic protein (BMP) family, both of which activate pathways essential for vascular in growth and odontogenic differentiation. DPSC-derived vesicles also contain dentinogenesis-associated microRNAs, including miR-21 and miR-218, which modulate Wnt, BMP, and other intracellular signaling networks fundamental to odontoblast maturation. Preclinical investigations demonstrate that these vesicles enhance dentin-like matrix deposition and promote the formation of vascularized pulp-like tissue, underscoring their translational promise for regenerative endodontic therapies (Ivica et al., 2021). The ready accessibility of DPSCs from extracted teeth and their high vesicle secretion capacity further strengthen their clinical applications. Additionally, the immunomodulatory effects of DPSC-derived vesicles help regulate inflammatory responses, establishing a microenvironment that supports orderly and predictable tissue repair.

6.3.2 Stem cells from the apical papilla

SCAP constitute another highly potent source of EVs with significant therapeutic value in regenerative endodontics. Positioned at the root apex of immature permanent teeth, SCAP exhibit rapid proliferation and a pronounced odontogenic phenotype. These cells are indispensable contributors to root maturation, dentin formation, and apexogenesis, making SCAP-derived vesicles particularly relevant for regenerative interventions in teeth with incompletely developed roots. SCAP-derived EVs possess a distinctive molecular profile enriched with BMP-2, VEGF, and neurotrophic mediators such as brain-derived neurotrophic factor. These factors act synergistically to promote odontoblast differentiation, stimulate neovascularization, and support neural regeneration, all of which are critical to the reconstitution of a functional pulp–dentin complex. The vesicles also contain regulatory microRNAs, including miR-140-5p, which modulate angiogenic and odontogenic pathways to enhance tissue repair. A hallmark feature of SCAP-derived vesicles is their capacity to drive apexogenesis and root elongation. Through the recruitment and differentiation of endogenous progenitor cells, these vesicles facilitate continued root development in cases of pulp necrosis, thereby addressing a major challenge in the management of immature teeth (Kong et al., 2023). Their strong proliferative potential and targeted molecular cargo make SCAP-derived vesicles a cornerstone of biologically centered treatment strategies for compromised young permanent teeth.

6.3.3 Periodontal ligament stem cells

PDLSCs, traditionally associated with periodontal tissue regeneration, have recently garnered attention as valuable contributors to pulp–dentin repair through their EVs. They are derived from the periodontal ligament, which is a specialized connective tissue anchoring the tooth to the alveolar bone. They exhibit considerable plasticity and multilineage differentiation potential, positioning them as an important alternative stem cell source for dental tissue engineering. EVs secreted by PDLSCs are enriched with ECM proteins, adhesion molecules, cytokines, and growth factors that orchestrate a range of regenerative processes. Their cargo includes potent pro-angiogenic mediators such as VEGF and interleukin-8, which stimulate endothelial proliferation and neovascularization, thereby supporting the metabolic demands of regenerating pulp tissue. The immunoregulatory capabilities of PDLSC-derived vesicles further modulate inflammatory cascades, limiting tissue damage and enhancing reparative outcomes. Although these stem cells are primarily involved in periodontal homeostasis, accumulating evidence indicates that their vesicles can also promote cell proliferation, matrix deposition, and structural restoration within the pulp–dentin complex. Consequently, PDLSC-derived vesicles broaden the repertoire of biologically relevant tools available for endodontic regeneration and underscore the versatility of dental mesenchymal stem cell-derived EVs in tissue repair.

6.4 DENTAL STEM CELL-DERIVED EVs IN PROMOTING PULP–DENTIN REGENERATION

Dental stem cell-derived EVs have shown remarkable potential in regenerative endodontics due to their unique biological properties and specialized molecular cargos. These vesicles serve as natural carriers of bioactive molecules, facilitating communication between cells and driving critical processes involved in pulp–dentin regeneration. Their unique attributes range from promoting odontogenic differentiation to immunomodulation, making them highly suited for addressing the challenges of dental tissue repair and regeneration.

6.4.1 Odontogenic potential

A defining feature of EVs derived from dental stem cells is their inherent capacity to drive odontogenic differentiation, a fundamental requirement for reparative dentin formation and the functional restoration of the pulp–dentin complex.

A. Growth Factors and Signaling Molecules: EVs derived from dental stem cells are enriched with a broad spectrum of growth factors, including members of the BMP family, transforming growth factor-beta (TGF-β), and insulin-like growth factors. These molecules are central to activating odontogenic signaling cascades such as the BMP/Smad and Wnt/β-catenin pathways, both of which are indispensable for odontoblast differentiation and dentin matrix synthesis. Among these mediators, BMP-2 and BMP-7 are particularly influential as they upregulate dentin-specific proteins including dentin matrix protein-1 and dentin sialophosphoprotein, key structural components required for the formation and mineralization of reparative dentin.

B. MicroRNAs (miRNAs): Dental stem cell-derived vesicles also transport a defined set of microRNAs, such as miR-21, miR-218, and miR-140-5p, that orchestrate odontogenic differentiation at the transcriptional and post-transcriptional levels. miR-21, for example, enhances the expression of dentin matrix protein-1 and dentin sialophosphoprotein, thereby promoting mineral deposition within the dentin matrix. These miRNAs additionally regulate transcription factors including Runx2, a master regulator governing both osteogenic and odontogenic lineage commitment, further reinforcing their central role in dentinogenesis.

C. Extracellular Matrix Proteins: EVs from dental stem cells also contain ECM proteins such as fibronectin, laminin, and collagen. These matrix components support cell adhesion, migration, and early lineage specification, providing a biomimetic scaffold that mimics the native ECM of the pulp–dentin complex. By offering structural and biochemical signals, these proteins facilitate organized dentin matrix deposition and contribute to the restoration of tissue architecture.

6.4.2 Angiogenic stimulation

Angiogenesis, the formation of new blood vessels from pre-existing vasculature, is a fundamental requirement for the successful regeneration of vital, functional pulp tissue. Adequate vascularization ensures the delivery of oxygen, nutrients, and signaling molecules necessary for cell survival, differentiation, and tissue homeostasis. EVs derived from dental stem cells have demonstrated strong pro-angiogenic activity, positioning them as key mediators in establishing a vascular network within the regenerating pulp–dentin complex.

A. Angiogenic Growth Factors: Dental stem cell-derived EVs transport a range of angiogenic growth factors, including VEGF, FGF, and platelet-derived growth factor. These molecules regulate distinct but complementary aspects of vascular development, from endothelial cell proliferation and migration to vessel stabilization. VEGF is particularly important for promoting capillary-like structure formation, whereas FGF contributes to the maturation and resilience of developing vascular networks.

B. MicroRNAs in Angiogenesis: In addition to growth factors, dental stem cell-derived vesicles carry angiogenic microRNAs such as miR-126 and miR-132, which modulate endothelial signaling at the post-transcriptional level. miR-126 enhances VEGF receptor activation and supports endothelial cell survival, thereby initiating vessel sprouting. miR-132 promotes the stabilization and integration of newly formed vessels by modulating pathways associated with endothelial maturation and pericyte recruitment.

C. Matrix Remodeling and Vessel Integration: EVs also contain matrix metalloproteinases (MMPs), which facilitate the controlled degradation of ECM components. This remodeling process enables endothelial cells to migrate and form new vascular structures within the dense matrix of regenerating pulp tissue. By coordinating matrix turnover with endothelial cell dynamics, vesicles promote efficient vascular integration and enhance the overall functionality of regenerated tissue.

6.4.3 Neurogenic support

Functional pulp regeneration requires the re-establishment of sensory innervation as nerves play essential roles in mediating pain perception, regulating blood flow, and coordinating reparative responses within the pulp–dentin complex. EVs derived from dental stem cells significantly contribute to neurogenesis and neural repair by delivering neurotrophic factors, regulatory microRNAs, and molecular cues that support neuronal survival and axonal integration.

A. Neurotrophic Factors: Dental stem cell-derived EVs are enriched with key neurotrophic mediators, including brain-derived neurotrophic factor, glial cell line-derived neurotrophic factor, and nerve growth factor. These molecules enhance neuronal viability, stimulate axonal extension, and promote synaptic maturation. Among them, brain-derived neurotrophic factor and nerve growth factor are particularly effective in supporting the regeneration of sensory nerve fibers, which are indispensable for maintaining pulp vitality and physiological responsiveness.

B. Neurogenic MicroRNAs: In addition to protein factors, these vesicles carry neurogenic microRNAs such as miR-124 and miR-9, which regulate gene networks involved in neuronal differentiation, axonal patterning, and neural circuit development. By influencing critical transcriptional programs, these microRNAs guide the formation and extension of regenerating nerve fibers, contributing to the structured re-innervation of the regenerated pulp tissue.

C. Functional Integration: Beyond promoting nerve outgrowth, dental stem cell-derived EVs facilitate the integration of regenerated nerve fibers into pre-existing neural networks. This functional incorporation restores sensory transmission and regulatory feedback mechanisms, which are crucial for a fully functional pulp. Successful neural integration establishes the physiological responsiveness of the regenerated tissue and represents a key benchmark for complete pulp regeneration.

6.4.4 Immunomodulation

The immune response exerts a critical and often paradoxical influence on tissue regeneration. While controlled inflammation is necessary to initiate repair, persistent or excessive immune activation can hinder healing and exacerbate tissue injury. EVs derived from dental stem cells demonstrate potent immunomodulatory capabilities, enabling them to shape the inflammatory milieu in ways that support predictable pulp–dentin regeneration (Figure 6.3).

A. Anti-Inflammatory Cytokines: Dental stem cell-derived EVs transport anti-inflammatory cytokines such as interleukin-10 and TGF-β. These cytokines suppress the expression of major pro-inflammatory mediators, including tumor necrosis factor-alpha (TNF-α) and interleukin-6, thereby attenuating early inflammatory responses and

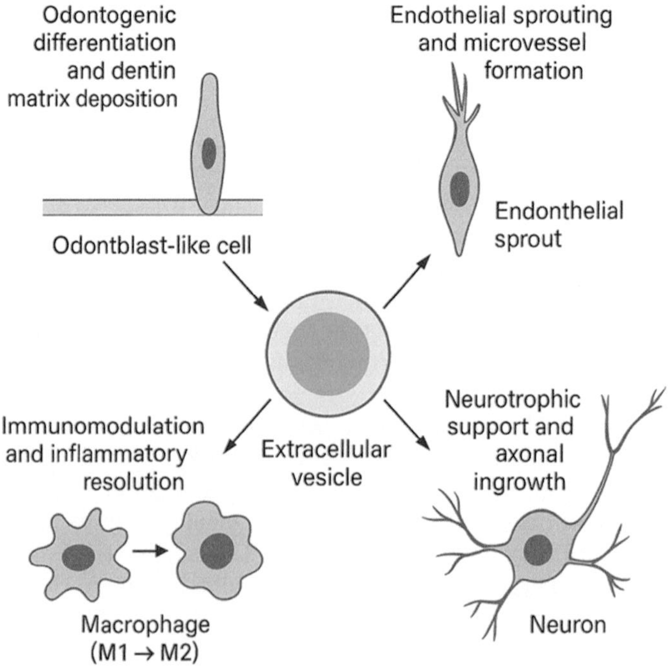

Figure 6.3 Mechanistic axes through which dental stem cell-derived extracellular vesicles support pulp–dentin regeneration. EVs from dental stem cells deliver growth factors, microRNAs, and matrix-associated proteins that promote odontoblast differentiation and reparative dentin deposition, stimulate endothelial sprouting and microvascular organization, enhance neural survival and axonal ingrowth, and shift macrophages from pro-inflammatory to reparative phenotypes.

preventing progression to chronic inflammation. This modulation helps preserve the structural and cellular integrity required for subsequent regenerative events.

B. Macrophage Polarization: A key mechanism underlying the immunoregulatory effects of these vesicles is their ability to influence the macrophage phenotype. Vesicle-associated factors promote a shift from the pro-inflammatory M1 phenotype toward the reparative M2 phenotype. M2 macrophages secrete anti-inflammatory mediators and ECM components that collectively enhance wound healing, limit tissue destruction, and support the early phases of pulp–dentin regeneration.

C. MicroRNAs in Immunomodulation: Dental stem cell-derived EVs also carry microRNAs such as miR-146a and miR-21, which target central inflammatory pathways, including NF-κB signaling. By downregulating key transcriptional drivers of inflammation, these microRNAs contribute to the resolution of inflammatory responses and help establish a microenvironment conducive to cellular proliferation, matrix deposition, and tissue repair.

6.4.5 Matrix remodeling and tissue integration

Matrix remodeling and tissue integration are essential processes in successful pulp–dentin regeneration. The ECM provides both the structural framework and biochemical cues that guide key cellular functions, including adhesion, migration, proliferation, and lineage commitment. EVs derived from dental stem cells play a central role in orchestrating these events by delivering molecular cargo capable of modifying the ECM and facilitating the incorporation of regenerated tissues into the native pulp–dentin architecture. Through the coordinated action of enzymes, matrix proteins, and adhesion molecules, these vesicles contribute to establishing a microenvironment conducive to stable and functional tissue regeneration.

6.4.6 Role of EVs in ECM remodeling

Matrix remodeling encompasses both the controlled degradation of damaged or necrotic ECM components and the synthesis and organization of new matrix proteins necessary for restoring tissue integrity. Dental stem cell-derived EVs participate directly in this remodeling process by transporting key molecules that regulate matrix turnover and structural renewal.

A. Matrix Metalloproteinases: EVs from DPSCs and SCAP are enriched with MMPs such as MMP-2 and MMP-9. These enzymes degrade denatured matrix components, including collagen and fibronectin, thereby clearing a path for progenitor cell migration and enabling the deposition of a newly synthesized ECM. The regulated enzymatic activity of MMPs is crucial for creating space within the tissue scaffold while preventing uncontrolled matrix destruction, ensuring a balanced remodeling response that supports regeneration.

B. Tissue Inhibitors of Metalloproteinases (TIMPs): In parallel with MMPs, dental stem cell-derived EVs also contain TIMPs, which modulate MMP activity and prevent excessive matrix degradation. The dynamic interplay between MMPs and TIMPs is essential for maintaining the structural integrity of the regenerating pulp–dentin complex. By stabilizing newly deposited matrix proteins and preventing premature breakdown, TIMPs contribute to the proper organization and maturation of the ECM.

C. Collagenases and Elastases: In addition to MMPs and their regulators, EVs carry collagenases, elastases, and related enzymes that selectively degrade specific matrix components. This targeted breakdown allows the replacement of compromised or necrotic matrix elements with newly synthesized proteins, facilitating progressive tissue repair and integration. The selective nature of this remodeling ensures that structural renewal occurs efficiently and in a controlled manner, supporting the long-term stability of regenerated tissues.

6.4.7 Enhancement of ECM synthesis

While the controlled degradation of the damaged ECM is necessary to prepare the microenvironment for repair, the synthesis and organization of new matrix components are equally essential for restoring the structural and functional integrity of the pulp–dentin complex. Extracellular vesicles derived from dental stem cells play a significant role in directing this constructive phase of matrix remodeling by delivering key proteins and regulatory molecules that support matrix assembly, stability, and mineralization.

A. Extracellular Matrix Proteins: Dental stem cell-derived EVs transport structural matrix proteins such as collagen, laminin, and fibronectin, which are incorporated into the regenerating tissue. These proteins form a scaffold that facilitates cell adhesion, migration, and spatial organization. Fibronectin within vesicles is particularly important for enhancing cell–matrix interactions, contributing to the alignment and stabilization of newly formed tissues and promoting the maturation of the ECM.

B. Proteoglycans and Glycoproteins: Vesicles also contain proteoglycans, including decorin, and glycoproteins such as tenascin-C, both of which play integral roles in matrix assembly and mechanical resilience. Proteoglycans interact with and sequester growth factors, enabling their gradual release and enhancing their biological availability within the regenerating microenvironment. These molecules contribute to matrix organization, regulate collagen fibrillogenesis, and support the biomechanical properties of newly formed tissue.

C. Mineralization Proteins: Dental stem cell-derived EVs are enriched with mineralization-related proteins such as dentin sialophosphoprotein and dentin matrix protein-1. These proteins promote the nucleation and growth of hydroxyapatite crystals, a process fundamental to dentin mineralization. By facilitating crystal deposition and maturation, vesicles support the restoration of dentin structure and mechanical strength, contributing to the long-term functionality of regenerated tooth tissues.

6.4.8 Facilitation of cellular interactions

Matrix remodeling driven by EVs is intrinsically interconnected with the regulation of cellular interactions, which are essential for coordinated tissue integration during pulp–dentin regeneration. Through their diverse molecular cargo, dental stem cell-derived EVs help establish a microenvironment that supports effective cell–matrix and cell–cell communication, enabling the organized assembly of regenerating tissues.

A. Adhesion Molecules: Dental stem cell-derived vesicles transport a variety of adhesion molecules, including integrins, cadherins, and selectins, which enhance cellular attachment to the ECM. Integrins are particularly important as they transduce mechanical and biochemical signals from the matrix into intracellular signaling pathways that regulate cell migration, proliferation, and differentiation. This integrin-mediated communication ensures that cells respond appropriately to the evolving microenvironment, promoting organized tissue regeneration.
B. Cytokines and Chemokines: EVs also contain chemokines and cytokines, such as interleukin-8 and stromal cell-derived factor-1, which function as potent chemoattractants for progenitors and stem cells. These signaling molecules guide cellular migration into the regenerating pulp–dentin complex, ensuring adequate cellular infiltration and providing a coordinated foundation for ECM deposition, tissue maturation, and functional integration.
C. MicroRNAs (miRNAs): In addition to protein mediators, vesicles carry microRNAs like miR-29 and miR-124 that regulate genes involved in ECM remodeling and cell–matrix interactions. miR-29 modulates collagen synthesis and matrix turnover, while miR-124 influences cytoskeletal organization and cell motility. Together, these microRNAs help fine-tune the cellular responses required for stable integration of regenerating tissues into the existing pulp–dentin structure.

6.4.9 Promotion of tissue integration

Tissue integration denotes the seamless incorporation of regenerated structures into the existing pulp–dentin complex, ensuring mechanical coherence and functional continuity. EVs derived from dental stem cells play a central role in this process by guiding matrix organization, facilitating vascular and neural incorporation, and promoting the functional stabilization of newly regenerated tissues.

A. Alignment of Collagen Fibers: Dental stem cell-derived EVs promote the alignment and organization of newly synthesized collagen fibers in accordance with the native ECM. This structural alignment is essential for preserving the biomechanical properties of the pulp–dentin complex, ensuring that regenerated tissues exhibit appropriate tensile strength, elasticity, and spatial orientation.
B. Stimulation of Vascular and Neural Integration: For regenerated pulp tissue to function effectively, newly formed vasculature and nerve fibers must integrate with existing networks. Vesicles facilitate this integration through their cargo of pro-angiogenic and neurogenic molecules, including VEGF and brain-derived neurotrophic factor. These mediators support the ingrowth, branching, and stabilization of blood vessels and sensory nerves, thereby ensuring adequate nutrient delivery, metabolic support, and sensory functionality within regenerated tissues.
C. Mechanical and Functional Stability: By promoting ECM organization and enhancing cell–matrix and cell–cell interactions, dental stem cell-derived EVs contribute to the mechanical and functional stability of regenerated tissues. This structural reinforcement reduces the risk of tissue detachment, degradation, or functional decline over time and is essential for the long-term success and durability of regenerative endodontic therapies.

6.4.10 Molecular cargos of dental stem cell-derived EVs

EVs derived from dental stem cells owe their regenerative functionality to the diverse molecular cargos they transport. These cargos encompass regulatory microRNAs, signaling and structural proteins, membrane lipids, and cytokines, each contributing uniquely to the biological processes required for pulp–dentin regeneration. By packaging these molecules into a stable vesicular structure, EVs enable their targeted delivery to recipient cells, where they modulate transcriptional programs, activate key signaling pathways, and orchestrate cellular behaviors essential for tissue repair. The following sections delineate the major categories of EV cargo and their specific roles in mediating odontogenic differentiation, angiogenesis, neurogenesis, immunomodulation, and ECM remodeling during regenerative endodontics.

6.5 MICRORNAS AS KEY REGULATORS OF GENE EXPRESSION

MicroRNAs represent one of the most influential classes of bioactive molecules transported by dental stem cell-derived EVs. These short, non-coding RNAs modulate gene expression by binding to complementary sequences within the 3′ untranslated regions of target mRNAs, resulting in either transcript degradation or translational repression (Bartel, 2018). Their encapsulation within vesicles protects them from enzymatic degradation, allowing them to retain stability and exert regulatory effects during intercellular communication. Within regenerative endodontics, vesicle-associated microRNAs orchestrate a variety of cellular processes essential for tissue renewal, particularly those governing odontogenic differentiation, angiogenesis, and immunomodulation (Figure 6.4).

A. Odontogenic Differentiation: DPSC-derived vesicles are enriched with miR-21 and miR-218, two microRNAs central to odontoblast lineage commitment. miR-21 enhances the expression of dentin sialophosphoprotein and dentin matrix protein-1, both of which are important for mineralized dentin formation, whereas miR-218 promotes

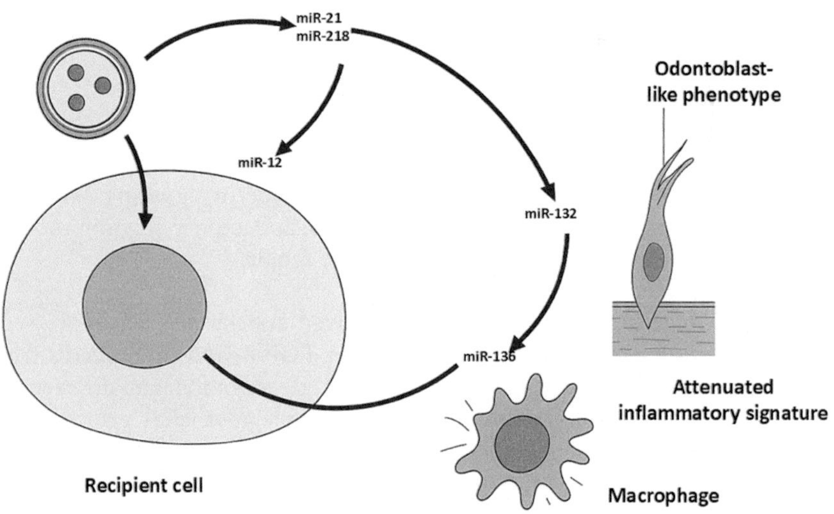

Figure 6.4 MicroRNAs within dental stem cell-derived EVs and their regenerative targets. EVs protect and deliver microRNAs that regulate key pathways in pulp–dentin repair. miR-21 and miR-218 enhance odontogenic differentiation by upregulating dentin matrix proteins and activating Wnt/BMP signaling. miR-126 and miR-132 augment angiogenesis by potentiating VEGF receptor signaling and stabilizing nascent vessels, whereas miR-146a attenuates NF-κB-driven inflammation, promoting a reparative immune milieu.

the Wnt/β-catenin signaling cascade, reinforcing the differentiation of progenitor cells into odontoblast-like cells capable of producing a mineralized matrix (Deng et al., 2015; Ivica et al., 2021).

B. Angiogenesis: Revascularization is critical for the survival and functionality of regenerated pulp tissue, and microRNAs such as miR-126 and miR-132 play central roles in this process. miR-126 amplifies VEGF receptor signaling in endothelial cells, stimulating their proliferation and motility, while miR-132 stabilizes nascent vessels by repressing anti-angiogenic pathways (Kong et al., 2023). Together, these microRNAs support the formation and maturation of a functional microvascular network.

C. Immunomodulation: MicroRNAs including miR-146a and miR-21 regulate inflammatory cascades by targeting key components of NF-κB signaling. Through this suppression, they reduce the synthesis of pro-inflammatory cytokines such as TNF-α and interleukin-6, thereby fostering a microenvironment conducive to tissue repair and limiting excessive inflammation (Sheedy, 2015). Through their ability to simultaneously influence multiple genes and pathways, vesicle-associated microRNAs serve as master regulators of the regenerative processes that underlie pulp–dentin repair, making them integral components of the therapeutic actions of EVs.

6.6 PROTEINS AS FUNCTIONAL MEDIATORS OF REGENERATION

Proteins constitute another major category of EV cargo and serve as direct mediators of regenerative activity. They participate in signaling cascades, structural remodeling, and ECM organization, collectively shaping the cellular environment in ways that support tissue repair.

A. Growth Factors: Dental stem cell-derived vesicles are rich in growth factors such as BMP-2, BMP-7, VEGF, TGF-β, and FGF. BMPs trigger Smad-dependent pathways that guide odontogenic differentiation, whereas VEGF and FGF coordinate endothelial proliferation and migration required for angiogenesis. TGF-β participates in both odontogenesis and immune regulation, promoting tissue stabilization and repair (Xuan et al., 2018; Liu et al., 2020).

B. Extracellular Matrix Proteins: Collagen, laminin, and fibronectin contained within vesicles provide structural scaffolds that facilitate cell adhesion and migration. These matrix proteins also contribute to the architectural organization and mechanical stability of newly forming tissue, ensuring the structural integrity of the regenerating pulp–dentin complex.

C. Enzymes and Regulatory Proteins: MMPs such as MMP-2 and MMP-9 assist in extracellular matrix remodeling by clearing damaged matrix components and generating space for new protein deposition. Additionally, regulatory proteins associated with Wnt and Notch signaling influence cell fate decisions and enhance stem cell differentiation, further supporting tissue regeneration (Mai et al., 2021). Protein cargos, therefore, act as multifunctional mediators that coordinate structural renewal, signaling events, and matrix remodeling, enabling a sustained and targeted influence on the regenerative microenvironment.

6.7 LIPIDS AS STRUCTURAL AND BIOACTIVE MOLECULES

Lipids contribute both structural stability and bioactive signaling functions to EVs. Their composition governs vesicle integrity, membrane fusion capability, and interactions with target cells, all of which are essential for effective cargo delivery.

A. Structural Lipids: Phospholipids including phosphatidylserine, phosphatidylcholine, and phosphatidylethanolamine form the foundational bilayer of vesicle membranes, ensuring mechanical stability and protecting internal cargos. Their distribution enhances vesicle fusion efficiency with recipient cell membranes and modulates uptake pathways (Subra et al., 2007).
B. Bioactive Lipids: Beyond structural roles, vesicular lipids such as sphingomyelin, ceramide, and eicosanoids act as potent signaling mediators. Ceramides facilitate endothelial migration and angiogenesis, supporting vascularization of regenerating pulp tissue, while eicosanoids, including prostaglandins, modulate inflammation and vascular permeability, thereby promoting a reparative microenvironment (Trajkovic et al., 2008). Through these combined attributes, lipids reinforce vesicle stability and actively contribute to the biological responses essential for tissue regeneration.

6.8 CYTOKINES AS MODULATORS OF IMMUNE RESPONSES

Cytokines packaged within dental stem cell-derived EVs are central to the regulation of inflammatory processes that dictate the trajectory of tissue repair. Their delivery in vesicular form ensures localized, controlled immunomodulation.

A. Anti-Inflammatory Cytokines: Cytokines such as interleukin-10 and TGF-β suppress the production of inflammatory mediators including TNF-α and interleukin-6, thereby limiting tissue damage and preventing chronic inflammation (Iyer and Cheng, 2012; Li et al., 2007; Saraiva et al., 2020). This targeted suppression enables a transition from early inflammatory phases to later reparative stages.
B. Chemokines: EV-associated chemokines like interleukin-8 and stromal cell-derived factor-1 act as chemoattractants that recruit progenitor and immune cells to the injury site. These molecules promote cellular infiltration, matrix deposition, and the coordinated assembly of regenerating tissue. Through their ability to regulate immune responses and direct cellular recruitment, cytokines within EVs establish a balanced immunological environment that supports effective pulp–dentin regeneration.

6.9 MOLECULAR ENGINEERING OF EXTRACELLULAR VESICLES FOR ENHANCED THERAPEUTIC POTENTIAL

EVs have gained increasing attention as a versatile platform for cell-free regenerative therapies, yet the therapeutic capabilities of naturally secreted vesicles are often limited by issues such as insufficient targeting specificity, rapid systemic clearance, and suboptimal loading of therapeutic molecules. Molecular engineering strategies aim to overcome these constraints by enabling precise modification of vesicle composition, surface architecture, and cargo. These approaches involve either engineering the parent cells that generate vesicles or implementing post-isolation modifications to fine-tune vesicle properties (Table 6.4). Through these methodologies, engineered vesicles achieve greater stability, enhanced tissue tropism, and improved therapeutic delivery, thereby expanding their potential for clinical translation. In the context of regenerative endodontics, such engineered vesicles offer the possibility of more efficient targeting of inflamed or damaged pulp tissues and improved orchestration of reparative processes.

Table 6.4 Engineering strategies to enhance EV therapeutic potential

Engineering strategy	*Mechanism/s*	*Benefits*
Genetic engineering	Overexpression of therapeutic miRNAs/proteins in parent cells	Enhances the regenerative capacity of EVs
Surface functionalization	Conjugation of targeting ligands (e.g., RGD peptides)	Improves tissue-specific delivery
Nanoparticle integration	Incorporation of gold/magnetic nanoparticles	Enables tracking and controlled release
Hydrogel encapsulation	EV embedding in biocompatible hydrogels	Sustained and localized therapeutic effect

6.10 GENETIC ENGINEERING OF EV-PRODUCING CELLS

Genetic manipulation of EV-producing cells represents a powerful strategy to refine the molecular composition and functional behavior of EVs. By introducing targeted genetic modifications into the parent cell, researchers can program the resulting vesicles to contain specific proteins, microRNAs, lipids, or targeting motifs, thereby enhancing their therapeutic efficacy. This ability to customize vesicle cargo and surface structure has significant implications for regenerative medicine, allowing the generation of vesicles tailored to induce precise biological responses within recipient tissues. The following subsections outline key strategies used to enhance targeting specificity, improve biodistribution, and prolong vesicle residence time.

6.10.1 Customizing surface proteins for targeted delivery

Among the most impactful advantages of genetic engineering is the ability to tailor EV surface proteins to improve targeting specificity. By manipulating the parent cell to express engineered ligands, peptides, or receptor-binding motifs on vesicle membranes, various vesicles capable of homing to defined cell populations or tissue microenvironments are generated.

A. Incorporation of Targeting Ligands: Genetic fusion of targeting ligands to vesicle-associated membrane proteins such as CD63, CD81, or Lamp2b enables precise surface presentation of functional peptides. A commonly used example involves fusing RGD peptide sequences to Lamp2b, enhancing vesicle binding to integrins that are upregulated in vascular or inflamed tissues. Such engineered vesicles exhibit improved tissue tropism and more selective therapeutic delivery, reducing off-target uptake and increasing therapeutic efficiency (Tian et al., 2014; Wang et al., 2017; Chen et al., 2021).
B. Cell-Specific Targeting: Tissue-specific peptides, single-chain antibodies, or receptor-binding motifs are genetically encoded in parent cells to produce vesicles with affinity for particular cell types. For instance, vesicles engineered to express epidermal growth factor ligands demonstrate enhanced uptake in epidermal growth factor receptor-positive cancer cells. Similar strategies could be adapted for regenerative endodontics, such as engineering vesicles to recognize receptors expressed on odontoblasts, DPSCs, or inflamed pulp tissues, thereby improving localized delivery of regenerative signals.
C. Immune-Evasion Markers: Genetic engineering is employed to incorporate immune-modulatory surface proteins, such as CD47, onto vesicle membranes. CD47 binds to signal regulatory protein α on macrophages, transmitting an inhibitory signal that suppresses phagocytic

activity and thereby prolongs vesicle persistence in circulation. Vesicles expressing CD47 or similar immune-evasion markers exhibit prolonged circulation times and improved biodistribution, thereby increasing their therapeutic availability *in vivo* (Kooijmans et al., 2016).

6.10.2 Optimizing cargo loading

Genetic engineering of EV-producing cells provides a powerful means of selectively enriching vesicles with therapeutic cargos such as microRNAs, proteins, and nucleic acid-based modulators. By altering the genetic profile of the parent cell, specific molecules can be preferentially packaged during vesicle biogenesis, allowing the generation of EVs with defined and enhanced regenerative properties.

A. miRNA Enrichment: Selective enrichment of microRNAs is particularly valuable given their central role in regulating pathways relevant to pulp–dentin regeneration. Overexpression of miR-21 and miR-218 in parent cells produces vesicles capable of strongly promoting odontoblast differentiation via activation of Wnt/β-catenin and BMP/Smad pathways (Deng et al., 2015; Kong et al., 2023). Similarly, engineering cells to overexpress miR-146a yields EVs with potent anti-inflammatory activity as these vesicles can suppress NF-κB signaling in inflamed pulp tissues, reducing cytokine expression and facilitating tissue repair.
B. Therapeutic Protein Loading: Genetic overexpression of therapeutic proteins in EV-producing cells results in vesicles enriched with growth factors and cytokines that act directly on recipient cells. Vesicles loaded with BMP-2 or BMP-7 stimulate odontogenic differentiation and promote reparative dentin formation, whereas those enriched with VEGF or FGF enhance vascular ingrowth and support metabolic activity within regenerating pulp tissue. This strategy ensures sustained, localized delivery of highly bioactive proteins.
C. Antisense RNA and siRNA Loading: Parent cells can also be engineered to package antisense RNAs or siRNAs into EVs, allowing targeted silencing of pathological genes in recipient cells. For example, vesicles carrying siRNAs against TNF-α reduce inflammation in pulpitis models, improving the microenvironment for tissue regeneration. This approach enables precise modulation of deleterious gene expression and supports controlled resolution of inflammatory processes.

6.10.3 Engineering EVs for multimodal applications

Genetic engineering enables the creation of multifunctional vesicles that integrate therapeutic, targeting, and diagnostic capabilities within a single platform. Such multimodal vesicles can simultaneously deliver diverse cargos, enhance targeting specificity, and permit real-time tracking of their biodistribution.

A. Therapeutic and Imaging Cargos: By expressing fluorescent proteins or radioactive reporters in parent cells, vesicles can be engineered to carry imaging markers alongside therapeutic agents. These modified EVs allow visualization of vesicle trafficking and tissue accumulation, enabling real-time assessment of therapeutic activity *in vivo*.
B. Dual or Multiplexed Therapeutic Loading: Genetic modification can be used to package multiple therapeutic cargos within the same vesicle. For example, EVs engineered to contain both anti-inflammatory cytokines (such as IL-10) and odontogenic proteins (such as dentin sialophosphoprotein) can simultaneously suppress inflammation and promote dentin regeneration. Such dual-action vesicles offer a comprehensive therapeutic strategy for pulp–dentin repair.
C. Integration with Biomaterials: Another emerging approach involves engineering EVs to display binding motifs that enhance their association with biomaterial scaffolds. Parent cells can be modified to express peptide sequences that bind hydrogels or ECM biomaterials, ensuring that vesicles remain localized at the treatment site and provide sustained therapeutic action over time.

6.10.4 Applications in regenerative endodontics

Genetically engineered EVs have significant potential to advance regenerative endodontics by enabling precise, targeted, and multifunctional therapeutic delivery. Through surface engineering and cargo customization, these vesicles can be directed to damaged pulp tissues, where they deliver regenerative signals with high specificity.

EVs engineered to express odontoblast-specific ligands can enhance targeted delivery of growth factors or microRNAs to dental pulp cells, thereby amplifying dentinogenic activity. Vesicles enriched with miR-21 or BMP-2 promote differentiation of DPSCs into odontoblast-like cells, accelerating reparative dentin formation. Similarly, EVs carrying anti-inflammatory payloads such as miR-146a or TGF-β can selectively target inflamed pulp tissues, that reduces inflammatory mediators and establishing a microenvironment conducive to regeneration. Through genetic engineering, EVs can be tailored to deliver these therapeutic cargos precisely where they are needed, minimizing systemic exposure and off-target effects. In addition, enrichment of EVs with pro-angiogenic and neurogenic mediators such as VEGF and brain-derived neurotrophic factor enhances vascularization and neural integration within the regenerating pulp–dentin complex. This comprehensive combination of targeted delivery, immunomodulation, and functional tissue integration underscores the transformative potential of engineered EVs for long-term restoration of pulp vitality.

6.11 SURFACE FUNCTIONALIZATION OF EXTRACELLULAR VESICLES

Beyond genetic modification of parent cells, direct surface functionalization has emerged as a complementary strategy for enhancing vesicle targeting, stability, and therapeutic performance. One widely explored approach involves the conjugation of targeting ligands to vesicle membranes. For example, the attachment of RGD peptides, which is known for their strong affinity to integrins expressed in the angiogenic vasculature, substantially improves site-specific EV delivery (Li et al., 2018). Advances in click chemistry further enable efficient, bio-orthogonal conjugation of functional molecules to EV surfaces without disrupting membrane integrity, allowing the incorporation of diverse targeting moieties (Smyth et al., 2014; Smyth et al., 2014; Lee et al., 2018). Hybrid nanovesicle systems represent another important innovation. By incorporating nanoparticles into or onto EV membranes, researchers can confer additional functionalities. Magnetic nanoparticles introduce magnetically guided targeting, improving localization and therapeutic precision (Qian et al., 2021). Similarly, integration of gold nanoparticles imparts photothermal capabilities, enabling combined therapeutic and theranostic applications. These hybrid systems illustrate the expanding versatility of engineered vesicles as advanced delivery platforms in regenerative medicine and beyond.

6.11.1 Applications in regenerative medicine

Surface-functionalized EVs have demonstrated considerable promise across several domains of regenerative medicine. In neural tissue engineering, for example, vesicles modified with neural cell adhesion molecules have been shown to promote neuronal differentiation, axonal extension, and functional repair, offering new therapeutic avenues for neurodegenerative diseases and traumatic neural injuries. Beyond regenerative applications, surface-engineered vesicles have also been explored in the field of cancer diagnostics, where they facilitate the detection of tumor-specific biomarkers. Through the incorporation of affinity ligands or recognition motifs, these modified vesicles enable sensitive and selective biomarker profiling, supporting early cancer diagnosis and personalized therapeutic strategies (Ma et al., 2021). These advancements underscore the versatility of surface-functionalized EVs and highlight their potential for translation into clinical settings, including endodontic tissue regeneration.

6.12 ADVANCED CARGO LOADING TECHNIQUES FOR EXTRACELLULAR VESICLES

While naturally secreted EVs exhibit intrinsic regenerative and immunomodulatory functions, their endogenous cargo may not always align with specific therapeutic goals in regenerative endodontics. Advanced cargo-loading techniques offer the opportunity to customize vesicle content, enabling the incorporation of targeted molecules such as microRNAs, proteins, growth factors, and nucleic acid therapeutics. These strategies significantly expand the therapeutic versatility of EVs and are particularly valuable for addressing challenges associated with pulp–dentin regeneration, inflammation control, and functional tissue restoration.

6.12.1 Electroporation for enhancing nucleic acid delivery

Electroporation is one of the most widely used approaches for introducing nucleic acids into EVs. This method employs short, high-voltage electrical pulses to transiently disrupt the vesicular lipid bilayer, creating pores that permit the diffusion of charged molecules such as miRNAs and siRNAs into the vesicle lumen. Following cessation of the electrical field, the membrane rapidly reseals, entrapping the therapeutic cargo. In regenerative endodontics, electroporation has yielded promising results. Deng et al. (2015) demonstrated effective loading of miR-218 into DPSC-derived EVs, resulting in vesicles capable of enhancing odontoblast differentiation and promoting dentin matrix formation. miR-218-enriched vesicles upregulated key odontogenic markers such as dentin sialophosphoprotein, highlighting their utility in dentin repair. Similarly, electroporation has been used to incorporate siRNAs that target inflammatory mediators such as TNF-α and IL-6 into EVs, significantly reducing inflammatory signaling in pulpitis models and supporting tissue healing. Despite its effectiveness, electroporation carries limitations, including the potential for vesicle aggregation or cargo degradation when high voltages are used. Careful optimization of pulse strength, duration, and buffer conditions is therefore essential to maintain vesicle integrity and ensure the stability of sensitive therapeutic molecules.

6.12.2 Mechanical disruption: sonication and extrusion

Mechanical loading techniques, including sonication and extrusion, represent alternative strategies that facilitate cargo incorporation by transiently destabilizing the vesicular membrane. These approaches are particularly advantageous for loading larger or hydrophilic molecules that do not readily diffuse across the lipid bilayer. Sonication applies high-frequency acoustic energy to induce mechanical perturbation of the vesicle membrane. During this transient disruption, therapeutic molecules present in the surrounding medium diffuse into the vesicle interior. Upon cessation of sonication, the membrane reseals, entrapping the cargo. This method has been successfully used to load regenerative proteins such as TGF-β and BMP-2 into

EVs (Qian et al., 2021). Preclinical studies have shown that these growth factor-enriched vesicles enhance odontogenic differentiation of DPSCs and accelerate reparative dentin formation. Extrusion, in contrast, involves repeatedly forcing vesicles and therapeutic agents through nanoscale membrane filters under precisely controlled pressure. This process disrupts the vesicle membrane, allowing cargos to mix with vesicular components before spontaneous resealing occurs. Extrusion has been used effectively to load anti-inflammatory agents into EVs for the treatment of pulp inflammation (Kong et al., 2023), resulting in vesicles that reduce inflammatory cytokine levels and support tissue repair. Both sonication and extrusion are scalable, efficient, and compatible with a wide range of therapeutic cargos. However, because these methods may alter vesicle size distribution, membrane composition, or morphology, post-loading quality assessments such as nanoparticle tracking analysis and cargo retention studies are essential to ensure functional consistency.

6.13 BIOLOGICAL ENGINEERING: NATURAL CARGO LOADING DURING BIOGENESIS

Biological engineering leverages the intrinsic machinery of EV-producing cells to load therapeutic cargos during vesicle biogenesis, allowing precise and stable incorporation of bioactive molecules without compromising vesicle integrity. By genetically modifying parent cells to overexpress targeted miRNAs, growth factors, or anti-inflammatory mediators, these molecules are selectively sorted into maturing EVs through natural intracellular trafficking pathways. This strategy has yielded vesicles with enhanced regenerative efficacy. For example, cells engineered to overexpress VEGF release VEGF-enriched EVs that markedly enhance angiogenesis in regenerating pulp tissues (Kong et al., 2023), a process indispensable for revascularizing the pulp–dentin complex. Similarly, EVs enriched with odontogenic miRNAs such as miR-21 and miR-218 promote differentiation of DPSCs by activating Wnt/β-catenin and BMP/Smad signaling pathways, accelerating dentinogenesis and reparative tissue formation (Deng et al., 2015). Engineered EVs carrying anti-inflammatory cargos have also shown efficacy in reducing pro-inflammatory cytokines in pulpitis models, creating a microenvironment favorable for regeneration. Although biologically engineered EVs offer exceptional precision and natural loading efficiency, this approach requires sophisticated genetic manipulation, is time-intensive, and poses challenges for large-scale production. Scaling such systems demands specialized bioreactors and rigorous quality control, underscoring the need for continued technological innovation to enable widespread clinical deployment.

6.14 METHODS TO ENHANCE EV STABILITY AND CIRCULATION TIME *IN VIVO*

A major barrier to the clinical translation of EV-based therapies is their rapid clearance from circulation via immune recognition, renal filtration, and enzymatic degradation (Figure 6.5). In regenerative endodontics, where sustained delivery of angiogenic, immunomodulatory, and odontogenic factors is essential, strategies that prolong EV stability and residence time are critical. Approaches such as polymer coating, hydrogel encapsulation, and lipid stabilization have demonstrated substantial promise in improving vesicle durability and therapeutic persistence.

6.14.1 Polymer coating for enhanced circulation and stability

Polymer coating, particularly with polyethylene glycol (PEG), is one of the most widely adopted methods to prolong EV half-life and protect them from immune clearance. PEGylation generates a hydrophilic steric barrier on the vesicle surface, reducing opsonization and phagocytosis while preserving structural stability. In regenerative endodontics, PEG-coated EVs carrying BMP-2 or other reparative cargos exhibit improved bioavailability and sustained release, resulting in enhanced odontoblast differentiation and reparative dentin formation. PEGylated EVs demonstrate significantly extended circulation times compared to unmodified vesicles. Kooijmans et al. (2016) reported that PEG coating markedly improved *in vivo* retention

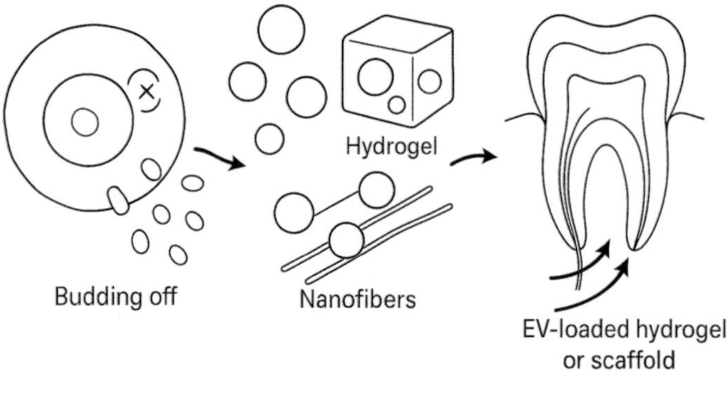

Figure 6.5 Translational engineering and delivery strategies for EVs in regenerative endodontics. Genetic modification of EV-producing cells, advanced cargo loading, and surface functionalization generate vesicles enriched with regenerative molecules and enhanced targeting properties. These engineered EVs can be integrated into hydrogels, nanofibrous scaffolds, or polymer-coated systems.

and therapeutic performance. However, potential immunogenicity with repeated administration remains a concern. Emerging alternatives such as zwitterionic polymers or biomimetic cloaking strategies may offer improved long-term biocompatibility.

6.14.2 Encapsulation in hydrogels for sustained localized delivery

Biodegradable hydrogels offer a robust platform for controlling EV release kinetics and protecting vesicles from premature degradation. Encapsulation within three-dimensional polymeric networks shields EVs from enzymatic breakdown while supporting gradual, sustained release at the target site. In pulp–dentin regeneration, hydrogel-encapsulated EVs enriched with VEGF or TGF-β have been shown to support angiogenesis and odontogenesis over extended durations (Kong et al., 2023). Hydrogels also allow tailoring of degradation profiles to clinical needs. The rapidly degrading systems suit acute injuries, while slower-degrading matrices support prolonged reparative phases. Challenges such as ensuring uniform vesicle distribution and preventing premature hydrogel degradation remain, though stimuli-responsive hydrogels that release EVs in response to environmental cues (pH and temperature) are promising innovations.

6.14.3 Lipid stabilization to improve structural integrity

Modifying the lipid composition of EV membranes can enhance vesicle mechanical strength and protect their cargo during systemic circulation. Incorporation of stabilizing lipids such as cholesterol or sphingomyelin increases membrane rigidity, reducing susceptibility to shear stress and enzymatic degradation. Lipid-stabilized vesicles have shown improved biodistribution and retention in regenerative tissues. Cholesterol-enriched EVs, for instance, display greater cargo retention and superior performance in inflammatory environments commonly encountered in pulpitis (Qian et al., 2021). This enhanced durability supports efficient delivery of fragile therapeutic molecules such as miRNAs. However, careful optimization is required to avoid excessive lipid loading, which may impact vesicle biocompatibility or induce undesirable immune responses.

6.15 IMMUNE EVASION FOR PROLONGING RETENTION TIME

Rapid immune-mediated clearance remains a major barrier to the sustained therapeutic activity of extracellular vesicles *in vivo*. Strategies that enable vesicles to evade recognition by phagocytic cells are, therefore, essential for prolonging circulation time and maximizing therapeutic delivery. One of the most effective approaches involves engineering EVs to display self-markers such as CD47, a transmembrane protein that interacts with signal regulatory protein-α on macrophages to inhibit phagocytosis. This interaction provides a potent immune-evasion signal that allows vesicles to persist longer within the host environment. In regenerative endodontics, where inflamed pulp tissues exhibit heightened immune activity, immune-evasive vesicles are particularly advantageous. EVs engineered to express CD47 have demonstrated markedly extended circulation times in inflammatory models, enabling sustained release of anti-inflammatory cargos to promote resolution of pulpitis. Simultaneously, these vesicles can be co-loaded with odontogenic factors such as BMP-7, ensuring that reparative processes proceed even in immunologically challenging microenvironments (Kamerkar et al., 2017). Despite their promise, several challenges remain, including the scalable production of CD47-engineered EVs and the need to mitigate potential off-target immune modulation. Advances in precise gene-editing technologies, including CRISPR-based engineering of donor cells, may enable the next generation of immune-evasive vesicles with improved safety, predictable behavior, and enhanced regenerative efficacy.

6.16 SUMMARY

EVs have emerged as a compelling cell-free therapeutic platform in regenerative endodontics, capable of coordinating the complex biological processes necessary for pulp–dentin repair. This chapter outlined the major EV subtypes and emphasized the distinctive regenerative potential of vesicles derived from dental stem cells, which deliver targeted cargos such as odontogenic growth factors, angiogenic mediators, neurotrophic molecules, ECM components, and regulatory miRNAs that collectively drive dentinogenesis, revascularization, neural repair, and controlled immunomodulation. Advances in EV engineering further expand their therapeutic utility. Approaches including PEGylation, hydrogel encapsulation, lipid stabilization, and biomaterial integration have enhanced EV stability, tissue retention, and localized cargo delivery. Complementary genetic and molecular engineering strategies now allow vesicles to be enriched with specific miRNAs, growth factors, or anti-inflammatory agents, enabling more precise and potent regenerative responses. Despite ongoing challenges such as standardizing isolation methods, ensuring scalable production, and validating clinical safety, EVs represent a significant step forward in developing predictable, biologically active therapies for endodontic regeneration. By bridging conventional cell-based approaches with next-generation bioengineering, EVs provide a promising, versatile platform for restoring pulp vitality and strengthening the foundation of regenerative dental medicine.

REFERENCES

Bartel, D. P. (2018). Metazoan microRNAs. *Cell*, 173(1), 20–51.

Chen, H., Wang, L., Zeng, X., Schwarz, H., Nanda, H. S., Peng, X., Zhou, Q., Li, N., & Ji, R. (2021). Exosomes, a new star for targeted delivery. *Frontiers in Cell and Developmental Biology*, 9, 751079.

Deng, Y., Zhou, H., Zou, D., Xie, Q., Bi, X., Gu, P., & Fan, X. (2015). The role of miR-218 in regulating differentiation of stem cells from apical papilla (SCAPs) into functional odontoblast-like cells. *Scientific Reports*, 5, 13952.

Gholami, L., Taghdiri Nooshabadi, V., Shahabi, S., Jazayeri, M., Tarzemany, R., Afsartala, Z., & Khorsandi, K. (2021). Extracellular vesicles in bone and periodontal regeneration: Current and potential therapeutic applications. *Cell & Bioscience*, 11(1), 59.

Ivica, A., Zehnder, M., & Weber, F. E. (2021). Therapeutic potential of mesenchymal stem cell-derived extracellular vesicles in regenerative endodontics. *eCM Journal*, 41, 252–263.

Iyer, S. S., & Cheng, G. (2012). Role of interleukin-10 in inflammatory lung diseases. *American Journal of Respiratory and Critical Care Medicine*, 185(5), 465–475.

Kamerkar, S., LeBleu, V. S., Sugimoto, H., Yang, S., Ruivo, C. F., Melo, S. A., Lee, J. J., & Kalluri, R. (2017). Exosomes facilitate therapeutic targeting of oncogenic KRAS in pancreatic cancer. *Nature*, 546(7659), 498–503.

Kong, H., Liu, P., Li, H., Zeng, X., Xu, P., Yao, X., Liu, S., Cheng, C. K., & Xu, J. (2023). Mesenchymal stem cell-derived extracellular vesicles: The novel therapeutic option for regenerative dentistry. *Stem Cell Reviews and Reports*, 19(1), 46–58. https://doi.org/10.1007/s12015-022-10342-y

Kooijmans, S. A. A., Fliervoet, L. A. L., van der Meel, R., Fens, M. H. A. M., Heijnen, H. F. G., van Bergen En Henegouwen, P. M. P., Vader, P., & Schiffelers, R. M. (2016). PEGylated and targeted extracellular vesicles display enhanced cell specificity and circulation time. *Journal of Controlled Release*, 224, 77–85.

Lee, T. S., Na, K., & Kim, H. (2018). Bio-orthogonally surface-engineered extracellular vesicles for targeted delivery. *Chemical Communications*, 54(78), 10976–10979.

Li, M. O., Wan, Y. Y., & Flavell, R. A. (2007). TGF-β regulation of immune responses. *Annual Review of Immunology*, 25, 435–472.

Li, S. P., Lin, Z. X., Jiang, X. Y., & Yu, X. Y. (2018, Apr). Exosomal cargo-loading and synthetic exosome-mimics as potential therapeutic tools. *Acta Pharmacologica Sinica*, 39(4), 542–551. https://doi.org/10.1038/aps.2017.178.

Liu, X., Yang, Y., Li, Y., Niu, X., Zhao, B., Wang, Y., Bao, C., Xie, Z., Lin, Q., Zhu, L., & Zhao, C. (2020). Integration of stem cell-derived exosomes with biomaterial scaffolds for tissue regeneration. *Stem Cell Research & Therapy*, 11, 194.

Ma, Y., Dong, S., Li, X., Kim, B. Y. S., Yang, Z., & Jiang, W. (2021). Extracellular vesicles: An emerging nanoplatform for cancer therapy. *Frontiers in Oncology*, 10: 606906.

Mai, Z., Chen, H., Ye, Y., Hu, Z., Sun, W., Cui, L., & Zhao, X. (2021). Translational and clinical applications of dental stem cell-derived exosomes. *Frontiers in Genetics*, 12, 750990.

Qian, X., Xu, C., Fang, S., Zhao, P., Wang, Y., Liu, H., & Yuan, W. (2021). Exosome-based nanocarriers: Preparation, drug loading, targeting, and delivery. *Acta Pharmaceutica Sinica B*, 11(7), 2092–2115. https://doi.org/10.1016/j.apsb.2021.01.020.

Saraiva, M., Vieira, P., & O'Garra, A. (2020). IL-10 and TGF-β: Two master regulators of immune tolerance. *Nature Reviews Immunology*, 20, 581–598.

Sheedy, F. J. (2015). Turning 21: Induction of miR-21 as a key switch in the inflammatory response. *Frontiers in Immunology*, 6, 19.

Smyth, T., Petrova, K., Payton, N. M., Persaud, I., Redzic, J. S., Graner, M. W., Smith-Jones, P., Anchordoquy, T. J., & Wang, M. (2014). Surface functionalization of exosomes using click chemistry. *Bioconjugate Chemistry*, 25(10), 1777–1784.

Subra, C., Laulagnier, K., Perret, B., & Record, M. (2007). Exosome lipidomics: A focus on lipid rafts and annexin-enriched domains. *Cellular and Molecular Life Sciences*, 64(17), 1967–1979.

Théry, C., Witwer, K. W., & Aikawa, E., Alcaraz, M. J., Anderson, J. D., Andriantsitohaina, R., Antoniou, A., Arab, T., Archer, F., & Atkin-Smith, G. K. (2018). Minimal information for studies of extracellular vesicles 2018 (MISEV2018): A position statement of the International Society for Extracellular Vesicles and update of the MISEV2014 guidelines. *Journal of Extracellular Vesicles*, 7(1), 1535750.

Tian, Y., Li, S., Song, J., Ji, T., Zhu, M., Anderson, G. J., Wei, J., Nie, Y., Niu, G., & Chen, X. (2014). A doxorubicin delivery platform using engineered natural membrane vesicle exosomes for targeted tumor therapy. *Biomaterials*, 35(7), 2383–2390.

Trajkovic, K., Hsu, C., Chiantia, S., Rajendran, L., Wenzel, D., Wieland, F., Schwille, P., Brügger, B., & Simons, M. (2008). Ceramide triggers budding of exosome vesicles into multivesicular endosomes. *Science*, 319(5867), 1244–1247.

Wang, J., Li, W., Lu, Z., Zhang, L., Hu, Y., Li, Q., Ge, Q., Lu, T., Ling, Y., Yu, H., & Wang, X. (2017). The use of RGD-engineered exosomes for enhanced targeting ability and synergistic therapy toward angiogenesis. *Nanoscale*, 9(45), 15598–15605.

Xuan, K., Li, B., Guo, H., Sun, W., Kou, X., He, X., Zhang, Y., Sun, J., Liu, A., Liao, L., Liu, S., Liu, W., Hu, C., Shi, S., & Jin, Y. (2018). Deciduous autologous tooth stem cells regenerate dental pulp after implantation into injured teeth. *Science Translational Medicine*, 10(455), eaaf3227.

Chapter 7

Immune response in regenerative endodontics

7.1 INTRODUCTION

Regenerative endodontics encompasses biologically guided therapeutic strategies that aim to restore the vitality, structural integrity, and functional capacity of the dentin–pulp complex. In contrast to conventional root canal therapy, which focuses primarily on the eradication of infection and the preservation of tooth structure, regenerative approaches seek to re-establish a physiologically active pulp environment characterized by cellular metabolism, vascular perfusion, and the capacity for continued dentin formation. Through this biologically centered framework, regenerative endodontics supports not only immediate tissue repair but also the long-term preservation of tooth vitality (Cooper et al., 2017). Central to this paradigm is the application of tissue engineering principles, which rely on the integrated action of three foundational components: stem cells, growth factors, and scaffolds. Stem cells derived from the apical papilla (SCAP) exhibit notable odontogenic potential, differentiating into odontoblast-like cells and contributing to dentin matrix deposition. Bioactive molecules such as transforming growth factor-beta (TGF-β) govern a wide range of cellular behaviors, including proliferation, chemotaxis, and lineage commitment, thereby directing the progression of tissue regeneration. Biomaterial scaffolds provide the three-dimensional framework necessary for these processes, supporting cellular organization, extracellular matrix (ECM) deposition, and controlled growth factor presentation to the developing tissues (Diogenes et al., 2019). Despite significant technological and biological advances, the predictability of regenerative endodontic procedures remains closely dependent on the host immune response. Immune activation is indispensable for initiating early repair events, including microbial clearance and recruitment of progenitor cells, yet excessive or prolonged inflammation can impair stem cell viability, alter signaling pathways, and disrupt scaffold integration. A nuanced understanding of immune-mediated modulation is, therefore, essential for optimizing regenerative outcomes and advancing next-generation endodontic therapies.

 DOI: 10.1201/9781003589921-7

7.2 THE IMPORTANT ROLE OF IMMUNE RESPONSES IN HEALING AND TISSUE REGENERATION

The immune system exerts a dual and highly regulated role in regenerative endodontics, functioning both as a frontline defense against microbial invasion and as a critical mediator of tissue repair. Following injury or infection of the dental pulp, innate and adaptive immune pathways are rapidly activated, initiating a cascade of molecular signals that recruit macrophages, dendritic cells, lymphocytes, and other effector cells to the site of damage (Table 7.1). These immune populations coordinate pathogen clearance, regulate early inflammatory events, and shape the microenvironment in which regenerative processes occur (Cooper et al., 2017). Macrophages are particularly central to these dynamics owing to their capacity to adopt distinct functional phenotypes in response to local signals. Classically activated M1 macrophages support antimicrobial defense and the initial inflammatory phase of wound healing, while alternatively activated M2 macrophages promote resolution of inflammation, ECM remodeling, and constructive tissue regeneration. Modulation of this M1–M2 continuum has emerged as a key determinant of regenerative success. Diogenes et al. (2019) demonstrated that intracanal medicaments and antibiotics used in regenerative protocols can alter macrophage polarization states, thereby influencing the biological trajectory of pulp–dentin repair. Beyond macrophages, cytokine networks play essential roles in regulating the balance between inflammation and regeneration. Pro-inflammatory mediators such as interleukin-1 beta (IL-1β), tumor necrosis factor-alpha (TNF-α), and interleukin-6 (IL-6) facilitate immune cell activation and recruitment, however, excessive or

Table 7.1 Key immune cells in regenerative endodontics

Immune cells	*Function*	*Role in regenerative endodontics*
Macrophages (M1)	Pro-inflammatory, antimicrobial activity	Initiates repair and clears pathogens but can delay regeneration if prolonged
Macrophages (M2)	Anti-inflammatory, tissue remodeling	Promotes healing, stem cell recruitment, and dentin–pulp regeneration
Neutrophils	First responders; pathogen clearance	Essential for early defense but may contribute to tissue damage if excessive
T-lymphocytes	Adaptive immunity and cytokine regulation	Regulates inflammation and modulates stem cell behavior
Dendritic cells	Antigen presentation and immune surveillance	Helps balance the immune response for controlled regeneration

prolonged exposure to these cytokines can impair stem cell differentiation into odontoblast-like lineages and disrupt tissue remodeling. In contrast, anti-inflammatory cytokines such as interleukin-10 help establish a reparative microenvironment by suppressing excessive inflammation and supporting the survival and function of resident and transplanted stem cells. The regenerative outcome, therefore, depends on the precise temporal coordination of these opposing immune signals, underscoring the intricate regulatory role of the immune system in endodontic tissue engineering. Moreover, the immune response exerts a direct regulatory influence on the behavior and regenerative capacity of stem cells involved in dentin–pulp restoration. Emerging evidence indicates that inflammatory signals can either enhance or suppress the odontogenic potential of stem cells, depending largely on the intensity, duration, and molecular composition of the signals. Transient, low-grade inflammatory stimulation has been shown to facilitate stem cell recruitment, promote chemotaxis, and prime odontogenic differentiation pathways. In contrast, persistent or excessive inflammation disrupts these processes, contributing to exhaustion of stem cells, impaired lineage commitment, and ultimately compromised regenerative outcomes. This context-dependent interaction highlights the necessity of controlling inflammation to support predictable and functionally integrated tissue regeneration (Figure 7.1).

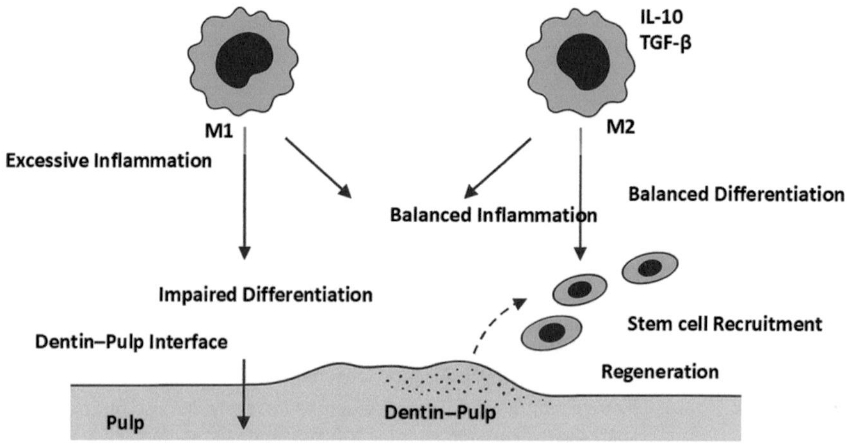

Figure 7.1 The figure illustrates the role of early inflammatory events in regulating pulp–dentin repair. M1 macrophages produce pro-inflammatory cytokines (IL-1β, TNF-α, and IL-6) that initiate antimicrobial defense but suppress stem cell differentiation when excessive. M2 macrophages release anti-inflammatory and reparative mediators (IL-10 and TGF-β), promoting stem cell recruitment, angiogenesis, and odontogenic differentiation.

7.3 INFLAMMATION AS A DOUBLE-EDGED SWORD IN ENDODONTIC REGENERATION

Inflammation constitutes a fundamental component of the host response to tissue injury and microbial invasion. Within the context of regenerative endodontics, this response functions as both a protective mechanism and a potential impediment to successful tissue regeneration. Acute inflammation, marked by the rapid influx of neutrophils, macrophages, and other immune effector cells, is essential for pathogen clearance and the establishment of a provisional microenvironment conducive to repair (Table 7.2). However, when the inflammatory response becomes prolonged or dysregulated, it can precipitate collateral tissue damage, promote fibrotic remodeling, and ultimately compromise the success of regenerative procedures (Cooper et al., 2017). The inherently dual nature of inflammation presents a major regulatory challenge for regenerative endodontics. Controlled, time-limited inflammation is indispensable for initiating reparative cascades, including the release of chemotactic and angiogenic factors and the recruitment of stem and progenitor cells to the site of injury. Conversely, persistent or excessive inflammatory signaling undermines these processes by inducing cytotoxicity, degrading ECM components, and suppressing the molecular pathways required for odontogenic differentiation. Diogenes et al. (2019) highlighted that precise modulation of inflammation is, therefore, central to the effectiveness of tissue engineering-based regenerative protocols,

Table 7.2 Inflammatory cytokines and their impact on regenerative endodontics

Cytokine	*Type*	*Function*	*Impact on regeneration*
Interleukin-1β (IL-1β)	Pro-inflammatory	Activates immune cells and promotes inflammation	Excessive levels hinder odontoblast differentiation
Tumor necrosis factor-α (TNF-α)	Pro-inflammatory	Enhances early immune response	High levels cause tissue destruction and stem cell apoptosis
Interleukin-6 (IL-6)	Pro-inflammatory	Mediates immune activation	Moderate levels enhance repair, and chronic elevation impairs healing
Interleukin-10 (IL-10)	Anti-inflammatory	Suppresses excessive inflammation	Supports tissue healing and promotes M2 macrophage polarization
Transforming growth factor-β (TGF-β)	Anti-inflammatory	Stimulates extracellular matrix formation	Promotes odontoblast differentiation and tissue repair

given its capacity to influence every stage of repair. Therapeutic strategies to manage inflammation in regenerative endodontics are continuing to evolve. Bioactive materials capable of locally releasing anti-inflammatory cytokines or modulating macrophage polarization have demonstrated potential in creating a microenvironment that supports constructive tissue regeneration. Likewise, certain antibiotics used in regenerative procedures not only reduce bacterial load but also modulate immune activity, illustrating their dual antimicrobial and immunoregulatory functions. Despite these advances, the mechanistic links between inflammatory mediators and regenerative outcomes remain incompletely understood. Future research will be essential to develop interventions that preserve the beneficial, initiation-phase aspects of inflammation while mitigating its deleterious chronic effects. Achieving this balance will be critical for optimizing the long-term success and predictability of regenerative endodontic therapies.

7.4 INTERPLAY BETWEEN INFLAMMATION AND REGENERATION IN THE DENTIN–PULP COMPLEX

Inflammation represents the body's immediate and essential response to injury or infection, functioning as a critical mechanism for neutralizing harmful stimuli and initiating reparative processes. Within the dentin–pulp complex, this reaction is highly regulated and involves a coordinated sequence of molecular and cellular events. Odontoblasts, which form the first line of defense at the pulpal interface, act as sentinel cells capable of detecting microbial invasion or physical insult (Table 7.3). Upon activation, odontoblasts secrete pro-inflammatory mediators such as IL-6, TNF-α, and various chemokines, which facilitate the recruitment of neutrophils, macrophages, T cells, and other immune populations to the site of injury (Hahn and Liewehr, 2007). The resulting inflammatory microenvironment initially not only amplifies host defense but also establishes the biochemical framework necessary for subsequent regenerative events. Importantly, the inflammatory milieu functions not only as a protective response but also as a preparatory phase for tissue regeneration. Bioactive molecules released during the early inflammatory phase promote the recruitment and activation of mesenchymal stem cells (MSCs) such as dental pulp stem cells (DPSCs) and SCAP. Moderate levels of pro-inflammatory cytokines have been shown to enhance the odontogenic differentiation of these stem cells, supporting the deposition of reparative dentin (Nakashima and Akamine, 2005). Concurrently, growth factors including vascular endothelial growth factor and TGF-β facilitate angiogenesis and ECM organization, both of which are essential for the functional restoration of pulp tissue. A notable advancement in recent years is the recognition that stem and progenitor cells derived from inflamed pulp retain substantial regenerative potential. Alongi et al.

Table 7.3 Modulation of inflammation by biomaterials in regenerative endodontics

Biomaterials	*Mechanism/s*	*Effect on immune response*	*Application in regenerative endodontics*
Bioactive glass	Ion release and surface mineralization	Reduces pro-inflammatory cytokines	Promotes dentin remineralization and stem cell attachment
Hydrogels (e.g., collagen and GelMA)	Provides ECM-like support	Modulates macrophage polarization	Supports pulp regeneration and stem cell migration
Calcium hydroxide	Alkaline pH; antimicrobial	Induces IL-10 and downregulates IL-6	Used in pulp capping to reduce inflammation
Scaffold-embedded growth factors	Sustained release of TGF-β and VEGF	Enhances wound healing	Encourages angiogenesis and dentinogenesis

(2010) demonstrated that these cells preserve their proliferation and differentiation capabilities despite exposure to inflammatory conditions, underscoring the adaptive resilience of dental stem cell populations. The temporal shift in macrophage polarization further illustrates how inflammation transitions into regeneration. Initial dominance of M1 macrophages supports antimicrobial defense and stem cell chemotaxis through the release of IL-1β and TNF-α. As healing progresses, a phenotypic shift toward M2 macrophages occurs, marked by the secretion of anti-inflammatory and reparative mediators such as IL-10 and TGF-β (Chapple and Matthews, 2021), thereby promoting matrix remodeling and tissue repair. Several molecular pathways integrate inflammatory signals with regenerative outcomes. The nuclear factor-kappa B (NF-κB) pathway plays a central role in regulating inflammatory gene expression and guiding stem cell recruitment. Similarly, the Wnt/β-catenin signaling axis has been shown to influence stem cell proliferation and differentiation in an inflammation-dependent manner, highlighting the intricate molecular crosstalk between immune activation and tissue regeneration (Haseeb et al., 2019). These insights carry significant therapeutic implications. Strategies aimed at modulating the inflammatory response can be leveraged to enhance regenerative outcomes. Controlled drug delivery systems incorporating bioactive scaffolds represent a promising approach, providing targeted release of anti-inflammatory agents and growth factors within the root canal environment. By fine-tuning inflammatory activity while preventing chronic or excessive responses, these technologies facilitate a microenvironment favorable for sustained and predictable regeneration. Collectively, the dual role of inflammation as both an initiator and regulator of tissue repair underscores its central importance in developing effective regenerative endodontic therapies.

7.5 CHRONIC INFLAMMATION AND ITS DETRIMENTAL EFFECTS

Chronic inflammation represents a pathological and sustained immune state that disrupts the delicate balance required for effective regeneration within the dentin–pulp complex. Unlike acute inflammation, which is self-limiting and functions to resolve injury and initiate repair, chronic inflammation is characterized by persistent immune activation and failure to transition toward resolution. This prolonged inflammatory state results in progressive tissue degradation, pulp necrosis, and the development of periapical pathosis, ultimately compromising the regenerative potential of the affected tissues (Rechenberg et al., 2016). Uncontrolled production of pro-inflammatory cytokines serves as a major driving force in this process, perpetuating immune cell activation, destabilizing tissue homeostasis, and generating a microenvironment that is fundamentally antagonistic to regeneration. Continuous secretion of mediators such as IL-1β, IL-6, and TNF-α impairs the biological functions of DPSCs. Under chronic inflammatory conditions, both the proliferative capacity and odontogenic differentiation potential of DPSCs are markedly reduced, a phenomenon associated with heightened oxidative stress and suppression of key odontogenic markers including dentin sialophosphoprotein (DSPP) and dentin matrix protein-1 (DMP-1) (Haseeb et al., 2019). This decline in stem cell function critically undermines the capacity of the pulp–dentin complex to mount an effective reparative response. The persistence of M1 macrophages is another hallmark of chronic inflammation. Failure to transition toward an M2-dominant reparative phenotype exacerbates tissue injury, disrupts ECM remodeling, and impairs angiogenesis, an essential component of pulp regeneration. Chronic inflammation also adversely affects the ECM by promoting fibrosis and dystrophic calcification, both of which impose physical and biochemical constraints on tissue repair. At the molecular level, aberrant activation of inflammatory signaling pathways further reinforces the chronic state. Overactivation of the NF-κB and mitogen-activated protein kinase (MAPK) pathways has been implicated in sustaining inflammatory gene expression, inhibiting regenerative cues, and promoting apoptosis or senescence in DPSCs (Zhang et al., 2015). These signaling alterations collectively diminish the tissue's ability to engage in constructive regeneration and reinforce the cycle of chronic disease. From a clinical perspective, effective management of chronic inflammation is crucial for restoring the regenerative capacity of the dentin–pulp complex. Anti-inflammatory therapies such as corticosteroids and nonsteroidal anti-inflammatory drugs (NSAIDs) may reduce inflammatory burden, though their use must be judicious to avoid impairing stem cell recruitment, proliferation, or differentiation. Emerging interventions, including targeted immunomodulatory agents, macrophage-polarizing strategies, and bioactive biomaterials capable of delivering controlled anti-inflammatory and pro-regenerative signals, hold significant promise for resolving chronic inflammation while preserving or restoring a microenvironment conducive to tissue regeneration.

7.6 MODULATION OF IMMUNE RESPONSES BY ANTIBIOTICS IN REGENERATIVE ENDODONTICS

In regenerative endodontics, effective control of microbial infection within the root canal system is foundational to creating a biologically favorable environment for tissue regeneration. While antibiotics have long been used for their antimicrobial efficacy, growing evidence indicates that they also exert significant immunomodulatory effects that influence both inflammatory and reparative phases of healing. This intersection between antimicrobial action, immune regulation, and tissue regeneration represents a promising yet complex therapeutic domain within regenerative endodontic therapy (RET) (Table 7.4). Over the past decade, research has increasingly elucidated how antibiotics affect key cellular activities, including macrophage polarization, stem cell viability, and biofilm disruption. Antibiotic therapy remains a principal component of regenerative endodontic procedures because of its broad-spectrum activity against the diverse polymicrobial communities found in the infected root canal system. The triple antibiotic paste (TAP), consisting of ciprofloxacin, metronidazole, and minocycline, is among the most extensively studied formulations. Designed to target both aerobic and anaerobic microorganisms, TAP effectively reduces the bacterial load that would otherwise impede tissue healing and regenerative signaling. Importantly, beyond their antimicrobial effects, antibiotics used in regenerative endodontics also influence host biological responses by modulating immune activity and shaping the inflammatory microenvironment.

Table 7.4 Impact of antibiotics on immune modulation in regenerative endodontics

Antibiotic	*Mechanism/s*	*Impact on immune cells*	*Effect on regeneration*
Ciprofloxacin	DNA gyrase inhibition	Reduces IL-1β and TNF-α	Suppresses inflammation and promotes repair
Metronidazole	Targets anaerobic bacteria	Inhibits oxidative stress and modulates cytokines	Supports healing, but high doses may impair stem cells
Minocycline	Anti-inflammatory and inhibits matrix metalloproteinases	Shifts macrophages to the M2 phenotype	Encourages regenerative environment
Amoxicillin-clavulanate	Broad-spectrum antibacterial	Minimal immune modulation	Primarily used for infection control

Ciprofloxacin, a representative fluoroquinolone, has been shown to exhibit immunomodulatory properties by altering cytokine production and macrophage function. Notably, it suppresses pro-inflammatory mediators including IL-1β and TNF-α, thereby supporting a microenvironment more conducive to tissue repair (Silva Lagos et al., 2022Kim). Metronidazole, an antiprotozoal and antibacterial agent, also contributes to immune regulation by inhibiting reactive oxygen species (ROS) formation, reducing oxidative stress-mediated damage during inflammation. Despite these therapeutic advantages, concerns remain regarding the cytotoxic effects of antibiotics on DPSCs and other progenitor cell populations essential for regeneration. High concentrations of TAP, although effective in microbial eradication, have been associated with reduced stem cell viability and impaired regenerative capacity (Zhang et al., 2015). These observations underscore the need for optimized antibiotic formulations and controlled delivery strategies that balance antimicrobial efficacy with preservation of stem cell function.

7.6.1 Impact of antibiotics on macrophage polarization and immune modulation

Macrophages are central regulators of both inflammation and tissue regeneration, and their functional plasticity enables them to assume distinct phenotypes that exert divergent biological effects. The two predominant polarization states, pro-inflammatory M1 macrophages and anti-inflammatory, pro-regenerative M2 macrophages, represent dynamic endpoints within a continuum shaped by local microenvironmental cues. Antibiotics commonly utilized in RET are now recognized as modulators of this polarization process. Experimental evidence demonstrates that agents such as ciprofloxacin can promote a phenotypic shift from M1 toward M2 macrophages, thereby facilitating the transition from an inflammatory to a reparative microenvironment. This shift is essential for resolving inflammation and initiating the cellular events required for tissue repair. M2 macrophages secrete key anti-inflammatory and pro-regenerative cytokines, including IL-10 and TGF-β, which play pivotal roles in recruiting and activating mesenchymal stem cells. Once activated, MSCs, including DPSCs and SCAP differentiate into odontoblast-like cells, contributing to dentin matrix deposition and overall tissue regeneration (Neves et al., 2020). A study published in the *Journal of Endodontics* further demonstrated that TAP reduces the synthesis of pro-inflammatory mediators while enhancing reparative signaling pathways in macrophages, highlighting the dual antimicrobial and immunomodulatory functions of antibiotics in RET. These findings underscore the therapeutic potential of antibiotics not only as agents to eliminate infection but also as modulators of immune cell behavior to improve regenerative outcomes (Figure 7.2). Nevertheless, the immunomodulatory effects of antibiotics are highly dose-dependent. Prolonged or excessive exposure may disrupt macrophage homeostasis, inhibit the appropriate

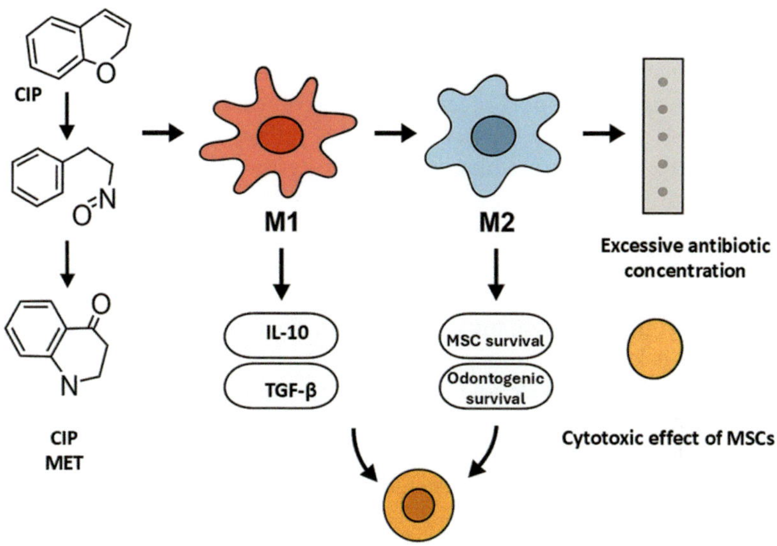

Figure 7.2 Immunomodulatory effects of antibiotics used in regenerative endodontics. The diagram illustrates how antibiotics such as ciprofloxacin and metronidazole influence macrophage polarization by suppressing pro-inflammatory cytokines (IL-1β and TNF-α) and enhancing anti-inflammatory mediators (IL-10 and TGF-β). This shift toward the M2 phenotype promotes stem cell survival and odontogenic differentiation. Excessive antibiotic concentration, however, exerts cytotoxic effects on stem cells.

transition to reparative phenotypes, or contribute to chronic inflammation, thereby compromising healing. A precise understanding of dosage, exposure duration, and formulation is, therefore, critical for optimizing RET protocols and ensuring predictable, biologically favorable outcomes.

7.6.2 Impact of antibiotics stem cell viability and differentiation

The viability and differentiation capacity of stem cells, particularly DPSCs and SCAP, are central determinants of successful RET. These stem cell populations contribute to the regeneration of the pulp–dentin complex by differentiating into odontoblast-like cells that synthesize dentin matrix components, including DSPP and DMP-1. Antibiotics employed in RET exert both beneficial and detrimental effects on stem cell biology, depending on the concentration, exposure duration, and specific formulation. At low concentrations, antibiotics such as ciprofloxacin and metronidazole have been shown to enhance stem cell differentiation by modulating inflammatory and reparative signaling pathways. These agents can upregulate odontogenic markers and augment the secretion of key growth factors, including vascular endothelial growth factor and TGF-β, both of which are critical for angiogenesis, ECM synthesis, and overall tissue repair (Iohara et al., 2011). Such findings highlight the potential of carefully calibrated antibiotic dosing to support regenerative outcomes. In contrast, higher concentrations of antibiotics, particularly minocycline, a component of the traditional TAP, demonstrate dose-dependent cytotoxicity that impairs stem cell proliferation and limits differentiation potential. This observed cytotoxicity has stimulated interest in alternative formulations in which minocycline is substituted with lower-toxicity antibiotics, such as amoxicillin or clindamycin, thereby supporting stem cell survival while retaining sufficient antimicrobial activity. (Zhang et al., 2015). Furthermore, the influence of antibiotics on key molecular pathways such as NF-κB and Wnt/β-catenin underscores their complex role in regulating stem cell behavior. Although these pathways are essential for stem cell activation and lineage commitment, excessive antibiotic-induced modulation can disrupt signaling balance, reinforcing the need for targeted, evidence-based therapies.

7.6.3 Role of antibiotics on biofilm disruption and enhanced disinfection

The presence of bacterial biofilms within the root canal system represents a major barrier to successful regenerative endodontics. Biofilms exhibit pronounced resistance to antimicrobial agents due to their dense extracellular polymeric matrix, reduced metabolic activity of resident bacteria, and the collective protective mechanisms afforded by structured microbial communities. Effective disruption of these biofilms is, therefore, essential to lowering the microbial and antigenic burden that perpetuates chronic inflammation and impedes tissue regeneration. Antibiotics remain central to this process. Ciprofloxacin and metronidazole have demonstrated substantial efficacy in biofilm disruption, with studies showing their capacity to penetrate the biofilm matrix and eradicate embedded bacterial populations. Recent advances have focused on enhancing antibiotic effectiveness against biofilm-associated infections. Nanoparticle-based delivery systems have emerged as a promising approach, improving both penetration and sustained retention of antimicrobial agents within the biofilm architecture. These systems increase local antimicrobial activity while limiting systemic exposure and toxicity (Fulaz et al., 2019). Beyond their direct antimicrobial properties, antibiotics also exert immunomodulatory effects in the context of biofilm-associated inflammation. By reducing the production of pro-inflammatory cytokines and promoting macrophage-mediated clearance of biofilm components, antibiotics help shift the local environment from a pro-inflammatory state toward one supportive of repair. This dual antimicrobial and immunoregulatory action contributes to the creation of a microenvironment conducive to pulp–dentin regeneration.

7.6.4 Immunotherapy as a potential strategy for vital pulp treatment

Vital pulp therapy (VPT) is a minimally invasive clinical strategy designed to preserve the vitality, structural integrity, and functional capacity of the dental pulp following exposure or traumatic injury. Conventional VPT procedures such as direct pulp capping and partial pulpotomy aim to protect the pulp by establishing a biocompatible barrier and stimulating reparative dentin formation. While these techniques have demonstrated substantial clinical success, their primary focus has traditionally been on providing structural protection rather than actively regulating the complex inflammatory and immune processes that govern pulp healing and long-term regenerative outcomes (Table 7.5). Recent advances in immunotherapy offer a transformative expansion of VPT by enabling targeted modulation of the host immune response. By leveraging the innate capacity of the immune system to resolve inflammation, promote angiogenesis, and support progenitor cell activation, immunomodulatory strategies have the potential to significantly enhance the biological efficacy of pulp preservation therapies. Incorporating controlled immune modulation into VPT represents a promising direction for achieving more predictable, biologically integrated, and durable regenerative outcomes.

7.6.4.1 Role of the immune system in pulpal healing

The dental pulp is a highly vascularized, richly innervated connective tissue enclosed within the rigid confines of dentin, rendering it particularly susceptible to inflammatory injury caused by caries progression, trauma, or operative procedures. Upon pulp exposure or insult, the innate immune system is rapidly activated, initiating the release of pro-inflammatory cytokines, chemokines, and other signaling mediators. This early inflammatory response functions as a critical host defense mechanism, promoting the recruitment of neutrophils, macrophages, and T lymphocytes to the site

Table 7.5 Immunotherapeutic approaches in vital pulp therapy

Approach	*Mechanism*	*Benefits in endodontics*
Cytokine modulation (IL-10 and TGF-β delivery)	Enhances M2 macrophage response	Reduces inflammation and promotes dentinogenesis
Nanoparticle-based drug delivery	Sustained release of bioactive molecules	Ensures targeted therapy and reduces systemic effects
Stem cell-based immunomodulation	DPSCs secrete anti-inflammatory cytokines	Balances immune response and enhances tissue repair
Hydrogel-encapsulated anti-inflammatory agents	Gradual cytokine and drug release	Creates a controlled regenerative microenvironment

of injury. Although acute inflammation is essential for microbial control and the initiation of reparative pathways, excessive or persistent inflammation can lead to irreversible tissue damage, culminating in pulp necrosis. Macrophages play a central role in orchestrating both the inflammatory and reparative phases of pulpal healing. Their capacity to polarize into distinct functional phenotypes, pro-inflammatory M1 or anti-inflammatory and pro-regenerative M2, is a key determinant of tissue outcomes. M1 macrophages predominate during the initial inflammatory phase, producing cytokines such as IL-6 and TNF- α that facilitate pathogen clearance and debris removal. Successful resolution of inflammation requires a timely shift toward the M2 phenotype, which supports angiogenesis, ECM deposition, and reparative dentinogenesis. Given the central regulatory role of the immune system in pulpal healing, contemporary immunotherapy approaches aim to modulate these immune responses to create a microenvironment optimized for tissue preservation and regeneration. By influencing cytokine profiles, macrophage polarization dynamics, and progenitor cell activation, immunotherapeutic strategies hold significant promise for enhancing the biological efficacy of VPT.

7.7 IMMUNOTHERAPY APPROACHES IN VITAL PULP TREATMENT

Immunotherapy in VPT represents a significant advancement in biologically guided endodontic care, harnessing the intrinsic regulatory capacity of the immune system to enhance healing, modulate inflammation, and promote regeneration of the pulp–dentin complex. Unlike traditional VPT techniques that primarily focus on providing a mechanical barrier to protect exposed pulp tissue, immunotherapeutic strategies directly engage the cellular and molecular processes that govern pulpal healing. This shift toward biologically active intervention reflects rapid progress in understanding how immune modulation can be integrated into regenerative dental therapies. A central objective of immunotherapy in VPT is the precise regulation of inflammation. While the early inflammatory phase is indispensable for initiating host defense and recruiting reparative cell populations, uncontrolled or prolonged inflammation can result in irreversible tissue damage and necrosis. Immunotherapeutic approaches seek to optimize this balance by promoting timely resolution of inflammation and facilitating the transition from an inflammatory to a reparative microenvironment. Cytokine modulation forms the foundation of these strategies. Pro-inflammatory cytokines such as IL-1β and TNF-α orchestrate early immune activation. However, sustained activity of these mediators can compromise healing. Targeted inhibition using monoclonal antibodies or small-molecule inhibitors has demonstrated efficacy in attenuating inflammation and preserving pulp viability (Arora et al., 2021). In contrast, anti-inflammatory cytokines including IL-10 and TGF-β are essential for resolving inflammation and supporting tissue repair. These cytokines drive macrophage polarization toward the M2 phenotype, which promotes angiogenesis, ECM deposition, and recruitment of MSCs. Localized delivery of IL-10 or TGF-β has been shown in preclinical models to enhance pulpal healing and stimulate reparative dentinogenesis (Zhang et al., 2015). Emerging technologies are further advancing immunotherapy through targeted delivery systems based on biomaterials and nanotechnology. Nanoparticles, hydrogels, and other engineered scaffolds are being developed to deliver immunomodulatory molecules directly to the pulp, enabling sustained release, localized bioactivity, and minimal systemic exposure (Neves et al., 2020). Hydrogels loaded with IL-10, for example, have demonstrated the ability to reduce inflammation and enhance reparative dentin formation in experimental settings. Stem cell-based immunomodulation provides an additional dimension to these strategies. DPSCs exhibit innate immunoregulatory properties, including the secretion of anti-inflammatory and pro-reparative factors that modulate immune activity while simultaneously contributing to tissue regeneration. Integrating DPSCs into immunotherapeutic approaches therefore offers a dual mechanism of action, addressing both the inflammatory burden and the regenerative demands of the pulp (Iohara et al., 2011).

7.7.1 Advantages of immunotherapy in VPT

Immunotherapy offers distinct advantages over traditional approaches to VPT by directly targeting the biological mechanisms that govern pulpal healing and regeneration. Conventional procedures such as direct pulp capping or partial pulpotomy primarily aim to establish a mechanical barrier to protect the exposed pulp; however, they do not actively engage the underlying inflammatory and immune processes that dictate long-term treatment success. In contrast, immunotherapeutic strategies modulate these biological responses in a targeted and dynamic manner, enabling more predictable and biologically integrated outcomes. A key advantage of immunotherapy is its capacity to regulate, rather than simply suppress, inflammation. The inflammatory response is essential for initiating repair by recruiting immune cells, clearing microorganisms, and activating reparative signaling pathways. Nevertheless, if inflammation becomes excessive or prolonged, it can result in irreversible tissue damage. Immunotherapy seeks to calibrate this response, facilitating efficient resolution of inflammation and timely progression to the reparative phase. For example, administration of anti-inflammatory cytokines such as IL-10 reduces excessive inflammatory signaling while simultaneously enhancing angiogenesis and reparative tissue formation (Arora et al., 2021). Immunotherapy also promotes the recruitment and activation of endogenous stem cells, which are essential for regenerating the pulp–dentin complex. By modulating the immune microenvironment, immunotherapeutic agents create conditions favorable for stem cell survival, proliferation, and differentiation into odontoblast-like cells. TGF-β exemplifies this dual functionality, suppressing inflammation while stimulating odontogenic pathways, making it highly valuable within the context of VPT (Zhang et al., 2015). Another significant benefit of immunotherapy lies in its potential to reduce treatment failures associated with chronic inflammation or persistent microbial challenges. Whereas conventional VPT depends on the physical integrity of restorative materials, immunotherapy addresses the underlying biological drivers of disease, decreasing the likelihood of pulp necrosis and improving long-term outcomes. Advances in nanotechnology have further expanded the therapeutic potential of immunotherapy. Nanoparticles, hydrogels, and other engineered delivery systems enable targeted, localized, and sustained release of immunomodulatory molecules at the site of pulp injury, thereby enhancing therapeutic precision while minimizing systemic exposure and adverse effects. These innovations position immunotherapy as a more biologically responsive and effective alternative for managing pulpal injuries and promoting predictable regeneration (Neves et al., 2020).

7.8 SUMMARY

The chapter emphasizes that immune regulation is fundamental to the success of regenerative endodontics. Unlike conventional treatment approaches that rely primarily on microbial removal, regenerative strategies depend on coordinated interactions between stem cells, growth factors, scaffolds, and a precisely modulated immune response to restore the dentin–pulp complex. Central to these interactions is the equilibrium between pro-inflammatory and anti-inflammatory pathways, which ultimately determines whether tissue repair advances or becomes impaired. Macrophage polarization encapsulates this duality as M1 activity is necessary for early defense and recruitment of reparative cells, while a timely shift to the M2 phenotype is essential for angiogenesis, matrix deposition, and odontogenic differentiation. Similarly, cytokines such as IL-1β and TNF-α initiate repair but impair regeneration when expressed chronically, whereas IL-10 and related mediators promote resolution and support stem cell function. This chapter also underscores that therapeutic success depends on effectively regulating this immunological balance. Emerging approaches, including immunomodulatory biomaterials, cytokine-targeted therapies, and antibiotics with immune-modifying properties, show considerable potential in establishing a microenvironment conducive to regeneration. However, achieving precise and reliable control over inflammatory dynamics remains a central clinical challenge. Continued progress in regenerative endodontics will rely on advancing immune-focused interventions and refining the integration of tissue engineering elements, ultimately enabling more predictable and durable biological restoration of the dentin–pulp complex.

REFERENCES

Alongi, D. J., Yamaza, T., Song, Y., Fouad, A. F., Romberg, E. E., Shi, S., & Tuan, R. S. (2010). Stem/progenitor cells from inflamed human dental pulp retain tissue regeneration potential. *Regenerative Medicine*, 5(4), 617–631.

Arora, S., Cooper, P. R., Friedlander, L. T., Rizwan, S., Seo, B., Rich, A. M., & Hussaini, H. M. (2021). Potential application of immunotherapy for modulation of pulp inflammation: Opportunities for vital pulp treatment. *International Endodontic Journal,* 54(8): 1263–1274. https://doi.org/10.1111/iej.13524.

Chapple, I. L. C., & Matthews, J. B. (2021). The role of the immune response in dentin-pulp regeneration: Understanding macrophage polarization. *Frontiers in Immunology*, 12, 705175.

Cooper, P. R., Holder, M. J., & Smith, A. J. (2017). Inflammation and regeneration in the dentin-pulp complex: Net gain or net loss? *Journal of Endodontics*, 43(9), S47–S55. https://doi.org/10.1016/j.joen.2017.06.010

Diogenes, A., Ruparel, N. B., Shiloah, Y., & Hargreaves, K. M. (2019). Antibiotics used in regenerative endodontics modify immune response of macrophages to bacterial infection. *Journal of Endodontics*, 45(1), 63–67. https://doi.org/10.1016/j.joen.2018.10.012

Fulaz, S., Vitale, S., Quinn, L., & Casey, E. (2019). Nanoparticle–biofilm interactions: The role of the EPS matrix. *Trends in Microbiology,* 27(11): 915–926. https://doi.org/10.1016/j.tim.2019.07.004.

Hahn, C. L., & Liewehr, F. R. (2007). Innate immune responses of the dental pulp to caries. *Journal of Endodontics*, 33(6), 643–651.

Haseeb, M., Pirzada, R. H., Ain, Q. U., & Choi, S. (2019). Wnt signaling in the regulation of immune cell and cancer therapeutics. *Cells,* 8(11), 1380. https://doi.org/10.3390/cells8111380

Iohara, K., Imabayashi, K., Ishizaka, R., & Nakashima, M. (2011). Dental pulp regeneration with stem cells from human exfoliated deciduous teeth. *Journal of Endodontics*, 40(1), S29–S33.

Nakashima, M., & Akamine, A. (2005). The application of tissue engineering to regeneration of pulp and dentin in endodontics. *Journal of Endodontics*, 31(10), 711–718.

Neves, V. C., Babb, R., & Sharpe, P. T. (2020). Modulation of inflammatory pathways in regenerative endodontics. *Journal of Endodontics*, 46(9), 1178–1187.

Rechenberg, D. K., Galicia, J. C., & Peters, O. A. (2016). Biological markers for pulpal inflammation: A systematic review. *PLoS One*, 11(11), e0167289.

Silva Lagos, L., Luu, T. V., De Haan, B., Faas, M., & De Vos, P. (2022). TLR2 and TLR4 activity in monocytes and macrophages after exposure to amoxicillin, ciprofloxacin, doxycycline and erythromycin. *Journal of Antimicrobial Chemotherapy*, 77(11), 2972–2985.

Zhang, J., Zhu, L. X., Cheng, X., Lin, Y., Yan, P., & Peng, B. (2015). Promotion of dental pulp cell migration and pulp repair by a bioceramic putty involving FGFR-mediated signaling pathways. *Journal of Dental Research*, 94(6), 853–862. https://doi.org/10.1177/0022034515572020.

Chapter 8

Growth factors and signaling pathways in dental regeneration

8.1 INTRODUCTION

Dental regeneration is an evolving field that integrates concepts from stem cell biology, biomaterials science, molecular signaling, and tissue engineering to develop novel therapies for the repair and regeneration of damaged or lost dental tissues. Over the past decade, advances in three-dimensional (3D) organoids, scaffold-based tissue engineering, and molecular modulation have significantly improved our understanding of dental tissue regeneration. Unlike traditional restorative dental treatments that merely replace lost structures with synthetic materials, regenerative approaches aim to biologically restore the form and function of dental tissues, including pulp, dentin, periodontal ligaments, and cementum (Nakashima and Iohara, 2017). Growth factors play a fundamental role in modulating cellular behavior, influencing stem cell proliferation, differentiation, extracellular matrix (ECM) deposition, and tissue homeostasis. These bioactive molecules are responsible for activating key signaling pathways that dictate the fate of dental stem cells and orchestrate tissue regeneration (Mao and Mooney, 2015). Several growth factors, including bone morphogenetic proteins (BMPs), transforming growth factor-beta (TGF-β), vascular endothelial growth factor (VEGF), fibroblast growth factors (FGFs), and insulin-like growth factors (IGFs), have been extensively studied for their regenerative potential in pulp–dentin complex repair, periodontal regeneration, and alveolar bone reconstruction (Kim et al., 2012; Duncan et al., 2018; Jung et al., 2019). On a molecular level, these growth factors interact with intracellular signaling pathways such as the Wnt/β-catenin, BMP-Smad, PI3K/AKT/mTOR, Notch, Hedgehog, and MAPK/ERK pathways to regulate the differentiation of dental pulp stem cells (DPSCs), stem cells from the apical papilla (SCAP), and periodontal ligament stem cells (PDLSCs) into functional dental tissues (Zhao et al., 2020). These pathways not only control cell survival and differentiation but also modulate angiogenesis, neurogenesis, and immune responses, which are essential for the long-term success of regenerative dental therapies.

DOI: 10.1201/9781003589921-8

8.2 GROWTH FACTORS IN DENTAL REGENERATION

Growth factors are essential regulatory proteins that orchestrate cellular processes such as stem cell proliferation, differentiation, ECM deposition, angiogenesis, and immune modulation. In the context of dental tissue engineering, these molecules play a pivotal role in pulp regeneration, dentin formation, periodontal repair, and alveolar bone remodeling (Galler et al., 2016). The various growth factors that are involved in dental regeneration are summarized in the subsequent sections (Figure 8.1).

8.2.1 Bone morphogenetic proteins

BMPs are a group of growth factors within the TGF-β superfamily that are known for their pivotal roles in bone and cartilage development. They were known to induce ectopic bone formation and also have been identified as critical regulators in various developmental and regenerative processes,

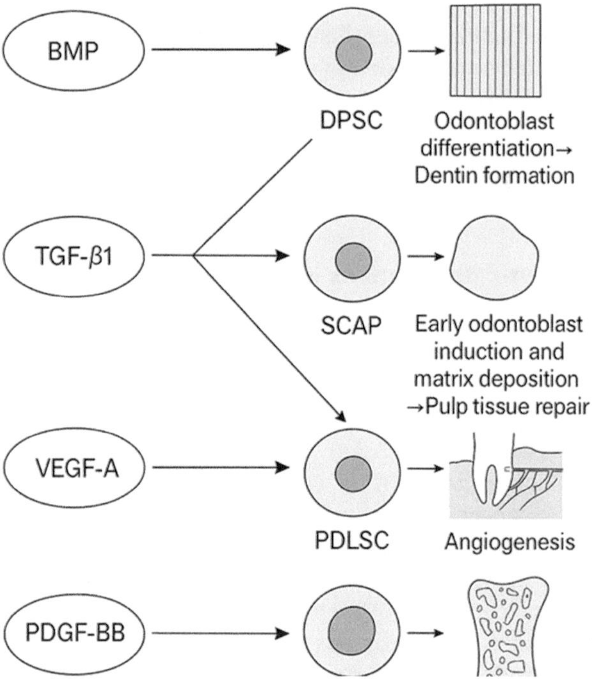

Figure 8.1 Major growth factors in dental regeneration and their cellular targets. Overview of key growth factors, namely, BMPs, TGF-β, VEGF, and PDGF, highlighting their primary actions on dental stem cell populations including DPSCs, SCAP, and PDLSCs. Stimulation by these growth factors drives lineage commitment toward pulp, dentin, periodontal ligament, and alveolar bone tissue regeneration.

including dental tissue formation and repair (Reddi and Huggins, 1972). During odontogenesis, BMPs are instrumental in the differentiation of dental mesenchymal cells into odontoblasts, the cells responsible for dentin formation. BMP-2, BMP-4, and BMP-7 have been extensively studied for their roles in tooth development. BMP-4, for instance, is expressed in the dental epithelium and influences the patterning and morphogenesis of teeth by regulating the expression of key transcription factors such as Msx1 and Msx2 (Vainio et al., 1993). BMP-2 and BMP-7 are involved in the differentiation of dental papilla cells into odontoblasts, promoting dentinogenesis (Nakashima and Reddi, 2003). BMPs exert their biological effects by binding to specific serine/threonine kinase receptors on the cell surface, known as BMP receptors type I and type II. Upon ligand binding, these receptors form heteromeric complexes, leading to the phosphorylation of receptor-regulated Smad proteins, including Smad1, Smad5, and Smad8. The phosphorylated Smads then form complexes with Smad4 and translocate into the nucleus, where they regulate the transcription of target genes that are involved in cell proliferation, differentiation, and ECM production (Miyazono et al., 2010).

In the context of dental tissues, BMP signaling promotes the expression of dentin matrix proteins such as dentin sialophosphoprotein (DSPP) and dentin matrix protein-1 (DMP-1), which are essential for the mineralization of dentin (Butler et al., 2003). Additionally, BMPs modulate the activity of other signaling pathways, including Wnt and FGF, to coordinate the complex processes of tooth development and regeneration (Liu and Millar, 2010).

8.2.1.1 Therapeutic applications in dental regeneration

The regenerative capacity of BMPs has been extensively explored across multiple domains of dental tissue engineering, with compelling evidence supporting their role in dentin pulp repair, periodontal regeneration, and alveolar bone augmentation. Their clinical utility, however, is moderated by critical challenges related to dosage, delivery, and cost, which continue to shape translational progress. In the context of dentin–pulp complex regeneration, BMP 2 has been widely examined as a biological alternative to traditional pulp-capping agents. Early studies demonstrated that exogenously applied BMP 2 effectively recruits and induces DPSCs to differentiate into odontoblast-like cells, promoting reparative dentin formation and preserving pulp vitality in cases of carious or traumatic exposure (Nakashima, 1994). Within periodontal engineering, BMP 7 has been employed to regenerate the alveolar bone-periodontal ligament-cementum complex. Clinical investigations have reported enhanced clinical attachment and improved bone fill in periodontal defects treated with BMP 7, underscoring its capacity to stimulate multilineage periodontal tissue repair (Giannobile et al., 1998). For alveolar ridge augmentation, BMP 2 is important due to its strong osteoinductive properties. Its application has been shown to induce robust bone formation within alveolar defects, thereby improving the structural basis for subsequent implant placement (Boyne et al., 2005). Despite this therapeutic promise, the clinical deployment of BMPs is constrained by several limitations. A major consideration is the dose-dependent nature of BMP signaling. While physiologically appropriate concentrations support controlled regeneration, excessive growth factor doses can trigger ectopic mineralization, heightened inflammatory responses, and abnormal differentiation patterns, underscoring the importance of stringent dose optimization (James, 2016; Zara et al., 2011; Oliveira et al., 2021). A parallel challenge lies in achieving effective and sustained local delivery. Multiple biomaterial platforms, such as collagen sponges, hydrogels, and synthetic polymer scaffolds, have been investigated to stabilize BMPs and modulate their release kinetics. Collagen-based carriers, for instance, permit gradual release of BMP 2 and have demonstrated efficacy in enhancing bone formation in periodontal defects (Jung et al., 2019). Additionally, the high cost of recombinant BMPs remains a significant barrier to widespread adoption. Emerging approaches aim to overcome this limitation by stimulating endogenous BMP expression, and gene-therapy-based delivery systems have shown promise in achieving localized, sustained BMP production without the need for repeated administration of recombinant proteins (Evans, 2011; Schwabe et al., 2012; Park et al., 2019). Together, these findings highlight both the established therapeutic value and the ongoing translational barriers associated with BMP-based interventions in dental regeneration. Continued refinement of dose control, delivery systems, and cost-effective production methods will be essential to fully realize their clinical potential.

8.2.2 Transforming growth factor-beta

TGF-β is a multifunctional cytokine that plays a pivotal role in regulating cellular processes such as proliferation, differentiation, apoptosis, and ECM production. In the context of dental tissues, TGF-β is sequestered within the dentin matrix and is released upon injury and influences the behavior of pulp cells and contributes to tissue repair and regeneration. TGF-β1, which is the most studied isoform in dental research, is integral to odontoblast differentiation and dentinogenesis. Upon dental injury, TGF-β1 is released from the dentin matrix, where it modulates the activity of DPSCs. Studies have demonstrated that TGF-β1 promotes the early differentiation of DPSCs into odontoblast-like cells, enhancing the expression of dentin matrix proteins such as DSPP and DMP-1 (Zhang et al., 2022). This process is crucial for the formation of reparative dentin, a natural defense mechanism of the tooth in response to the injury. Additionally, TGF-β1 has been shown to regulate the proliferation and osteogenic differentiation of DPSCs. A meta-analysis by Li et al. (2023) concluded that TGF-β1 significantly promotes the proliferation and ossification of DPSCs, indicating its potential in dental tissue engineering and regenerative therapies. TGF-β1 exerts its effects through both canonical (Smad-dependent) and noncanonical (Smad-independent) signaling pathways. Upon binding to its receptors on the cell surface, TGF-β1 activates receptor-regulated Smad proteins (Smad2 and Smad3), which then form complexes with Smad4. These complexes translocate into the nucleus to regulate the transcription of target genes involved in cell differentiation and ECM production (Moustakas and Heldin, 2009). In addition to the Smad pathway, TGF-β1 can activate other signaling cascades, including the MAPK, PI3K/AKT, and Rho-like GTPase pathways, which contribute to its diverse biological effects (Zhang, 2009). In dental pulp cells, TGF-β1 has been shown to activate the ERK1/2 pathway, promoting cell proliferation and differentiation (Zhang et al., 2022).

8.2.2.1 Therapeutic applications in dental regeneration

TGF-β1 is a central regulator of dental tissue homeostasis and repair, and its regenerative potential has been evaluated across several clinically relevant applications. Its ability to modulate odontoblast differentiation, matrix secretion, and stem cell behavior forms the basis of its therapeutic relevance in vital pulp therapy, dentin–pulp complex engineering, and craniofacial regeneration. In vital pulp therapy, TGF-β1 has been incorporated into bioactive pulp-capping strategies to stimulate reparative dentinogenesis. Experimental studies demonstrate that exogenous TGF-β1 promotes the differentiation of DPSCs into odontoblast-like cells and accelerates the deposition of a reparative dentin bridge, thereby maintaining pulp vitality following traumatic or carious exposure (Zhang et al., 2022). In tissue engineering contexts, TGF-β1 has been integrated into scaffold-based systems designed to regenerate the entire dentin–pulp complex. A notable approach involves photoactivation of endogenous latent TGF-β1 using low-power lasers, which induces *in vivo* dentin regeneration by directing the differentiation of resident dental stem cells and leveraging intrinsic biological reservoirs rather than exogenous protein delivery (Arany et al., 2014). Beyond the pulp, TGF-β1 also influences the activity of stem cells from human exfoliated deciduous teeth, enhancing their proliferation and osteogenic differentiation, thereby presenting additional opportunities for dental and craniofacial tissue engineering (Chang et al., 2020). However, the therapeutic application of TGF-β1 is limited by several biological and translational challenges. A primary concern is its propensity to induce fibrosis when present at excessive levels, resulting in abnormal ECM accumulation that can impair functional tissue regeneration. This underscores the requirement for precise modulation of its activity (Li et al., 2023). Effective clinical use also depends on developing delivery systems capable of stabilizing TGF-β1 and releasing it in a controlled manner within the target microenvironment.

Biomimetic scaffolds and engineered controlled release matrices are being explored to address these delivery constraints (Arany et al., 2014). Additionally, TGF-β1 engages in extensive signaling crosstalk with multiple molecular pathways, making its downstream effects context-dependent and sometimes unpredictable. Further mechanistic studies are required to clarify these interactions and inform rational therapeutic design.

8.2.3 Vascular endothelial growth factor

VEGF is a key regulator of angiogenesis, orchestrating the formation of new blood vessels from existing vasculatures and thereby sustaining the metabolic and defensive functions of dental tissues. Within the dental pulp, VEGF is indispensable for maintaining tissue vitality, supporting reparative responses, and enabling regeneration by ensuring an adequate and responsive vascular supply. Its expression contributes to oxygen and nutrient delivery, immune cell trafficking, and the overall homeostasis required for root formation and pulp defense. VEGF exerts its biological effects through binding endothelial cell receptors, primarily VEGFR1 and VEGFR2. Ligand engagement activates a series of intracellular signaling events that drive endothelial proliferation, migration, and the sprouting of new micro vessels. These processes are essential during both tooth development and post-injury responses, where enhanced angiogenesis facilitates reparative dentinogenesis and pulp healing following carious or traumatic insult. Notably, VEGF expression is consistently observed in both immature and mature pulps, highlighting its continuous physiological role. Higher expression levels of VEGF and its receptors in mature apex teeth suggest a compensatory mechanism to meet the heightened metabolic and immunological requirements of fully developed dental tissues. Signal transduction downstream of VEGF receptor activation prominently involves MAPK, ERK, and PI3K AKT pathways, which collectively promote endothelial cell survival, proliferation, and direct migration. VEGF also increases vascular permeability, enabling the extravasation of nutrients, progenitor cells, and immune mediators into the pulp microenvironment, an effect that becomes especially critical during tissue repair. In addition to VEGFRs, co-receptors such as neuropilin 1 further potentiate VEGF-mediated signaling, refining the spatial and temporal precision of angiogenesis within the pulp.

8.2.3.1 Therapeutic applications in dental regeneration

The pro-angiogenic activity of VEGF has been leveraged in multiple therapeutic strategies aimed at improving dental tissue regeneration. By promoting vascular growth and enhancing microcirculatory support, VEGF contributes directly to the survival, differentiation, and functional integration of regenerating tissues within the dental environment. In regenerative endodontic procedures, VEGF plays a central role in revitalizing necrotic pulp by promoting the angiogenic processes required for sustaining newly formed pulp-like tissue. Approaches that incorporate bioactive scaffolds and chemotactic growth factors rely on VEGF-mediated neovascularization to ensure adequate nutrient delivery, immune cell recruitment, and long-term tissue viability. Beyond its vascular effects, VEGF also modulates the behavior of DPSCs. Experimental studies demonstrate that DPSCs cultured in advanced platelet-rich fibrin-conditioned media show elevated VEGF A expression, which enhances their angiogenic capacity and supports both proliferation and differentiation. These findings emphasize the potential benefit of incorporating VEGF or VEGF-stimulating substrates into regenerative protocols to promote more robust tissue formation. A further challenge in dental tissue engineering is the insufficient vascularization of transplanted scaffolds, which limits the survival of implanted cells. Pre-vascularization strategies address this limitation by integrating endothelial cells and angiogenic factors such as VEGF into scaffolds prior to implantation, enabling rapid anastomosis with the host vasculature and improving the regenerative performance of engineered pulp and craniofacial tissues. Results from experimental models indicate that VEGF-enriched pre-vascularized constructs significantly enhance tissue survival and integration compared to nonvascularized constructs. Despite these benefits, the clinical translation of VEGF-based therapies remains constrained by several key considerations. Controlled delivery is a primary challenge as angiogenesis is highly sensitive to growth factor concentration. Supraphysiological levels may produce an abnormal or leaky vasculature, whereas inadequate delivery fails to support regeneration, necessitating the development of delivery systems capable of sustained, spatially controlled VEGF release. The selection of the VEGF source also influences the therapeutic efficacy. Autologous preparations such as platelet-rich fibrin (PRF) provide a natural supply of VEGF, but inherent variability in PRF composition and release kinetics underscores the need for standardized formulations. Additionally, VEGF acts within a complex regenerative milieu that involves multiple signaling molecules and growth factors. Understanding these interactions is crucial for designing combination therapies that effectively recapitulate the coordinated processes underlying natural tissue repair.

8.2.4 Platelet-derived growth factor

PDGF is a multifunctional mitogen that regulates key cellular processes including proliferation, migration, and angiogenesis, making it a promising therapeutic candidate in dental and periodontal regeneration. Among its various isoforms, PDGF BB is the most extensively investigated in oral tissue engineering due to its strong chemotactic and pro-regenerative properties. PDGF BB exerts its biological effects by binding to its cognate tyrosine kinase receptors, PDGFR α and PDGFR β, initiating intracellular signaling cascades that drive cellular activities essential for tissue repair. In periodontal tissues, PDGF BB has been shown to enhance the proliferation and directed migration of periodontal ligament cells, thereby contributing to the reconstruction of the periodontal ligament, cementum, and alveolar bone. Its capacity to stimulate angiogenesis further supports regeneration by improving vascular supply and promoting the metabolic and immune functions necessary for healing. Following receptor activation, PDGF BB triggers several downstream pathways, most notably the PI3K AKT and MAPK cascades. These signaling events promote cell survival, proliferation, and motility and induce the expression of genes associated with ECM synthesis and angiogenic regulation. Additionally, PDGF BB influences matrix dynamics by modulating integrin expression and regulating matrix metalloproteinases, thereby facilitating cell adhesion, matrix turnover, and coordinated tissue remodeling.

8.2.4.1 Therapeutic applications in dental regeneration

The regenerative potential of PDGF BB in dental tissues has been examined across a wide range of experimental and clinical models, reflecting its capacity to modulate cell recruitment, proliferation, angiogenesis, and matrix formation. Collectively, these investigations highlight PDGF BB as a key biological mediator capable of enhancing periodontal, peri-implant, and dentin–pulp regeneration. In periodontal regeneration, recombinant human PDGF BB has demonstrated significant clinical efficacy when delivered alone or in combination with bone graft materials. Clinical trials, including the landmark study by Giannobile and colleagues (1998), reported notable increases in bone fill and attachment level gain in periodontal defects treated with rhPDGF BB. These results establish PDGF BB as an effective stimulus for rebuilding periodontal structures involving the alveolar bone, periodontal ligament, and cementum. In the context of peri-implant bone regeneration, PDGF BB has been evaluated for its ability to enhance osseous healing around dental implants. Experimental evidence indicates that PDGF BB stimulates osteoblast proliferation and differentiation while simultaneously promoting angiogenesis, thereby improving early bone formation and increasing the stability of implants positioned in compromised or defect-containing sites. These combined osteogenic and angiogenic effects support the use of PDGF BB as an adjunctive agent in peri-implant regenerative therapies. Emerging data also suggest a potential role for PDGF BB in dentin–pulp complex regeneration. *In vitro* and *in vivo* studies demonstrate that PDGF BB enhances the proliferation and odontogenic differentiation of DPSCs, indicating its potential usefulness in regenerative endodontic protocols aimed at re-establishing the vitality, structure, and function of the dentin–pulp complex. Although research in this domain remains at an early stage, these findings point to additional clinical applications for PDGF BB beyond periodontal and osseous repair.

8.3 SIGNALING PATHWAYS

Signaling pathways constitute the fundamental regulatory networks that coordinate the cellular and molecular events driving dental tissue regeneration. They govern critical processes including stem cell proliferation, lineage differentiation, angiogenic activation, and ECM synthesis, all of which collectively support the restoration and functional reconstruction of dental structures (Figure 8.2).

8.3.1 Wnt/β-catenin signaling pathway

The Wnt β catenin signaling pathway is a fundamental regulatory axis governing cell proliferation, differentiation, and tissue homeostasis, and it plays an essential role in tooth development, maintenance, and repair. Activation of this pathway begins when Wnt ligands bind to frizzled receptors and the co-receptors LRP5 or LRP6 on the cell membrane. This ligand–receptor interaction inhibits the β catenin destruction complex, allowing β catenin to accumulate in the cytoplasm and subsequently translocate to

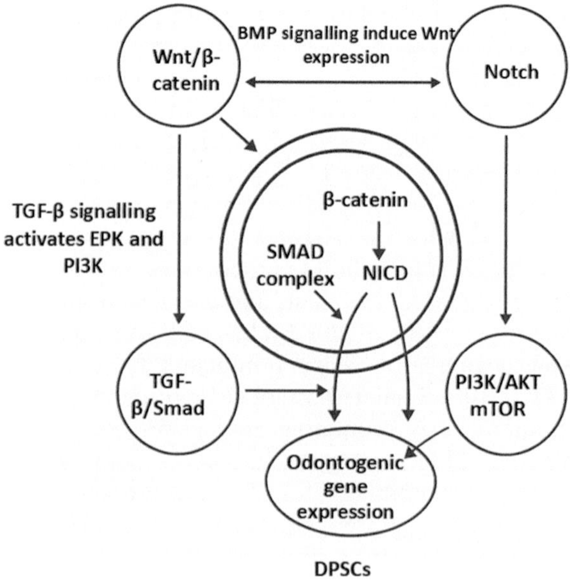

Figure 8.2 Crosstalk among key signaling pathways involved in odontogenic differentiation. Major pathways involved in dental tissue regeneration, including Wnt/β-catenin, BMP-Smad, TGF-β–Smad, PI3K/AKT/mTOR, and Notch signaling. Arrows illustrate pathway convergence on transcriptional regulation within DPSCs and highlight key interaction points that coordinate odontoblast differentiation and tissue repair.

the nucleus. Within the nucleus, β catenin associates with TCF LEF transcription factors to modulate the expressions of downstream genes involved in lineage specification and cellular proliferation (Clevers, 2006). During odontogenesis, Wnt β catenin signaling exhibits dynamic spatiotemporal regulation in both the dental epithelium and mesenchyme. The pathway is crucial for initiating tooth formation and for subsequent morphogenetic transitions. Experimental studies demonstrate that Wnt β catenin activation in the dental epithelium is required for dental placode formation, the earliest morphological hallmark of tooth development (Liu and Millar, 2010). Moreover, conditional deletion of β catenin in the dental mesenchyme leads to severe defects in tooth morphogenesis and differentiation, highlighting the indispensability of this pathway in odontogenic progression (Chen et al., 2009). In postnatal dental tissues, Wnt β catenin signaling continues to regulate the behavior of DPSCs. DPSCs, a mesenchymal stem cell population with odontogenic potential, respond robustly to canonical Wnt ligands. Activation of the pathway using Wnt3a enhances DPSC proliferation and upregulates key odontoblastic markers such as DSPP and DMP1, which correlates with increased mineralization capacity (Zhang et al., 2016). This demonstrates that Wnt β catenin signaling serves as a potent driver of odontoblastic differentiation. Odontoblast maturation is intricately controlled through multiple interacting signaling pathways, with Wnt β catenin functioning as a primary modulator. Sustained activation promotes the expressions of genes associated with terminal odontoblast differentiation and dentin matrix synthesis. Conversely, pathway inhibition disrupts these processes. The application of Wnt antagonists such as DKK1 leads to marked reductions in DSPP expression and impaired mineral deposition, underscoring the requirement of canonical Wnt activity for proper odontoblast differentiation and dentinogenesis (Yamashiro et al., 2007). Wnt/β-catenin signaling does not operate in isolation but interacts with other pathways to coordinate dental tissue regeneration. Notably, there is crosstalk between Wnt and BMP signaling pathways during odontogenesis. Studies have indicated that BMP2 can induce the expression of Wnt ligands, thereby activating Wnt/β-catenin signaling, which in turn promotes odontoblast differentiation (Liu et al., 2013). Additionally, the interplay between Wnt/β-catenin and Notch signaling pathways has been implicated in the regulation of DPSC proliferation and differentiation, suggesting a complex network of signaling interactions governing dental regeneration (Blokzijl et al., 2003). The crucial role of Wnt/β-catenin signaling in dental regeneration has significant therapeutic implications. Modulation of this pathway offers a promising strategy for enhancing reparative processes in dental tissues. For instance, the application of Wnt agonists has been explored to stimulate the regenerative capacity of DPSCs in pulp-capping procedures, aiming to promote the formation of reparative dentin and preserve pulp vitality (Neves et al., 2017). Moreover, tissue engineering approaches utilizing scaffolds incorporated with Wnt ligands or mimetics have been investigated to facilitate the regeneration of the dentin–pulp complex (Kim et al., 2012).

8.3.2 Transforming growth factor-beta signaling

TGF-β is a central regulatory cytokine that governs dental tissue development, homeostasis, and regeneration. It influences odontoblast differentiation, dentin matrix synthesis, ECM remodeling, and the behavior of DPSCs. TGF-β signals through both SMAD-dependent and SMAD-independent mechanisms and coordinate diverse cellular processes that are critical for maintenance of pulp–dentin complex and repair. Canonical signaling is initiated when TGF-β binds to its type II receptor, which recruits and phosphorylates the type I receptor. This activates receptor-regulated SMADs, primarily SMAD2 and SMAD3, which form a complex with SMAD4 and translocate to the nucleus to regulate genes that control proliferation, differentiation, and matrix production. In parallel, noncanonical pathways, including MAPK cascades such as ERK, JNK, and p38, as well as PI3K AKT signaling, contribute to cytoskeletal dynamics, stress responses, and inflammatory modulation. TGF-β is also involved in odontoblast differentiation and dentinogenesis. It upregulates the expressions of dentin-specific proteins, including DSPP and DMP-1, that are essential for mineralization. DPSCs exposed to TGF-β exhibit enhanced odontogenic differentiation and increased mineral deposition, confirming its role in promoting dentin matrix formation. In the dentin matrix, TGF-β is sequestered in a latent form and released following injury. Once released, it orchestrates the recruitment of stem cells to the injury site and promotes their differentiation into odontoblast-like cells, thereby initiating and sustaining reparative dentinogenesis. This mechanism is important following pulp exposure or traumatic insult, where TGF-β facilitates dentin bridge formation and contributes to pulp preservation.

The interaction between TGF-β and DPSCs has important implications for regenerative endodontics. Exposure to TGF-β enhances DPSC proliferation, chemotaxis, and differentiation, supporting pulp–dentin complex reconstruction. Tissue engineering strategies incorporate TGF-β into biomaterials to exploit these properties. Hydrogels and fibrin-based scaffolds that are enriched with TGF-β have shown the ability to promote pulp-like tissue formation, while bioactive glass and calcium silicate-based materials used in vital pulp therapy release endogenous TGF-β, further stimulating reparative responses and promoting pulp vitality. TGF-β operates within a highly integrated signaling milieu, interacting with numerous developmental pathways to coordinate cellular responses. Its interaction with Wnt β catenin signaling contributes to coordinating the balance between stem cell proliferation and lineage commitment, thereby ensuring controlled odontoblast differentiation during both development and tissue repair. In addition, TGF-β acts synergistically with Notch signaling to refine odontogenic lineage specification and maintain tissue homeostasis. Together, these intersecting regulatory networks underscore the necessity for precise spatial and temporal modulation of TGF-β activity to achieve consistent and predictable regenerative outcomes.

Therapeutic modulation of TGF-β signaling is being actively explored to enhance pulp–dentin regeneration. The scaffolds that are enriched with TGF-β have demonstrated considerable potential for regenerating the entire pulp–dentin complex. Further clinical studies suggest that TGF-β releasing biomaterials can effectively stimulate reparative dentinogenesis in direct pulp-capping procedures. However, translating these findings into clinical practice remains challenging due to the need for precise control over TGF-β activity. Excessive or prolonged signaling can induce fibrosis or dystrophic calcification, thereby undermining functional regeneration. Moreover, inter-individual variation in responsiveness to TGF-β-based interventions highlights the importance of personalized or adaptive therapeutic approaches. Future research should prioritize the design of delivery systems capable of achieving finely controlled release kinetics and the detailed elucidation of TGF-β's interactions with other signaling pathways, thereby optimizing its therapeutic application in regenerative endodontics.

8.3.3 Notch signaling pathway

The Notch signaling pathway is a highly conserved juxtacrine communication system that regulates cell proliferation, differentiation, and lineage specification across a wide range of developmental and homeostatic contexts. Within dental tissues, Notch signaling plays an important regulatory role in controlling the behavior of DPSCs and influences their capacity to differentiate into odontoblast-like cells that are required for dentin formation. Notch receptors (Notch1–4) are single-pass transmembrane proteins that are activated only upon direct cell-to-cell contact with their ligands, including Delta-like (Dll1, Dll3, and Dll4) and Jagged (Jag1 and Jag2) proteins. Ligand engagement triggers sequential proteolytic cleavages that release the Notch intracellular domain, which translocates to the nucleus and regulates transcriptional cascades that are involved in cell maintenance and differentiation. Current evidence indicates that Notch signaling plays a key role in maintaining DPSCs in an undifferentiated and proliferative state. Experimental overexpression of Jagged1 inhibits odontoblastic differentiation, indicating that active Notch signaling can preserve stemness while suppressing the odontogenic differentiation. In contrast, inhibition of Notch signaling promotes DPSC differentiation toward an odontoblast-like phenotype and enhances dentin matrix production. Notch signaling also contributes to the regulation of angiogenesis within regenerating pulp tissues. Biomaterials engineered to modulate Notch activity, including Notch signaling hydrogels, have shown the capacity to support rapid vascularization and promote pulp tissue regeneration, underscoring the pathway's broader involvement in establishing a microenvironment conducive to repair. Importantly, Notch does not function as an isolated regulatory mechanism. It intersects with multiple signaling pathways that are relevant to dental regeneration, including Wnt β catenin and TGF-β pathways. These interactions add complexity to the regulation of DPSC behavior and highlight the integrated nature of signaling networks that govern odontogenic differentiation and tissue regeneration.

8.3.4 Bone morphogenetic protein signaling

BMPs are a subgroup of growth factors within the TGF-β superfamily and serve as key regulators of proliferation, differentiation, and apoptosis. In dental regeneration, BMP signaling plays an essential role in tooth development, particularly in odontoblast differentiation and dentin formation, and remains central to the regenerative potential of DPSCs. BMP signaling is initiated when BMP ligands bind to heteromeric complexes of type I and type II serine threonine kinase receptors on the cell surface. Ligand binding induces phosphorylation of the receptor-regulated SMADs (SMAD1, SMAD5, and SMAD8), which subsequently associate with SMAD4 and translocate to the nucleus to regulate the transcription of genes that regulate the odontogenic differentiation and dentin matrix synthesis. In addition to this canonical pathway, BMPs activate noncanonical signaling cascades, including MAPK pathways, which cooperate with SMAD signaling to modulate cellular responses that are relevant to dental tissue regeneration. During tooth development, BMP signaling is indispensable for the differentiation of odontoblasts. BMP2 has been shown to promote odontogenic differentiation of human dental pulp cells by activating the Wnt β catenin signaling pathway, an effect partially mediated through p38 MAPK, indicating functional crosstalk between BMP and Wnt pathways during odontoblast maturation. BMP4 also contributes to dentinogenesis by regulating odontoblast differentiation and the expression of downstream dentin-related genes. In dental tissue engineering, BMPs have been extensively investigated for their ability to enhance the regenerative capacity of DPSCs. BMP7 promotes DPSC migration and odontogenic differentiation and supports angiogenic processes that are critical for pulp tissue regeneration. The utility of BMPs further extends to periodontal regeneration. Both BMP2 and BMP7 have demonstrated the capacity to induce the differentiation of progenitor cells into osteoblasts and cementoblasts, thereby contributing to the restoration of alveolar bone, periodontal ligament, and cementum. Recent advances have explored the modulation of BMP antagonists as an alternative means of enhancing endogenous BMP activity. Inhibition of USAG 1, a known BMP antagonist, has been shown to potentiate BMP signaling and induce *de novo* tooth formation in murine models, highlighting the therapeutic promise of targeting BMP regulatory networks to promote dental tissue regeneration.

8.3.5 PI3K/AKT/mTOR signaling

The phosphoinositide 3 kinase AKT (PI3K AKT) mammalian target of rapamycin signaling pathway is a central regulator of proliferation, survival, metabolism, and differentiation. In dental tissues, this pathway contributes to the regulation of odontogenic differentiation in a manner that appears to be highly dependent on the cellular context and microenvironmental signals. Several studies indicate that attenuation of PI3K AKT activity can favor odontogenic differentiation. Autophagy-mediated inactivation of the PI3K AKT pathway has been shown to enhance the odontogenic commitment of dental pulp cells by maintaining stemness at early stages while permitting subsequent differentiation. Similarly, suppression of the AKT mTOR branch increases the osteogenic and dentinogenic potential of SCAP, suggesting that reduced pathway activity can facilitate lineage progression in certain progenitor populations.

In contrast, other investigations report that active PI3K AKT signaling supports the proliferation, migration, and odontogenic differentiation of DPSCs. Pharmacological inhibition of the pathway leads to reduced DPSC proliferation and motility, together with downregulation of odontogenic markers, indicating that pathway activation may be necessary for specific phases of odontoblast maturation. These divergent findings indicate that the PI3K AKT mTOR pathway does not exert a uniformly promotive or inhibitory effect on odontogenic differentiation. Instead, its influence appears to vary depending on the developmental stage of the cells, the presence of growth factors, matrix signals, and interactions with other pathways such as MAPK or Wnt. Clarifying how these variables shape PI3K AKT mTOR signaling outputs will be essential for defining how this pathway can be targeted to enhance regenerative outcomes in dental tissues.

8.4 CONCLUSION

The integration of growth factors and signaling pathways into regenerative strategies has fundamentally advanced the field of dental tissue restoration, shifting the focus from conventional replacement toward biologically guided repair. Key growth factors, including BMPs, TGF-β, VEGF, and PDGF, regulate stem cell behavior and orchestrate the formation of dentin, pulp, periodontal ligament, and alveolar bone. Concurrently, molecular pathways such as Wnt β catenin, BMP-Smad, and PI3K AKT mTOR coordinate the proliferation, differentiation, and matrix synthesis required for predictable tissue regeneration. Despite these advances, important challenges persist, particularly in achieving controlled spatiotemporal delivery of bioactive molecules, mitigating risks such as fibrosis or ectopic mineralization, and translating experimental approaches into clinically feasible therapies. Emerging developments in biomaterial-based delivery platforms, gene modulation strategies, and precision medicine offer promising avenues to overcome these limitations. Continued investigation into the interactions and regulatory hierarchies among these pathways will be essential for refining and optimizing regenerative approaches. As the field progresses, the transition of biologically driven dental regeneration from experimental research to clinical practice will open new possibilities for restoring dental tissues with greater fidelity and long-term functional success.

REFERENCES

Arany, P. R., Cho, A., Hunt, T. D., Sidhu, G., Shin, K., Hahm, E., Huang, G. X., Weaver, J., Chen, A. C.-H., Padwa, B. L., Hamblin, M. R., Barcellos-Hoff, M. H., & Kulkarni, A. B. (2014). Photoactivation of endogenous latent transforming growth factor–β1 directs dental stem cell differentiation for regeneration. *Science Translational Medicine*, 6(238), 238ra69. https://doi.org/10.1126/scitranslmed.3008234

Blokzijl, A., Dahlqvist, C., Reissmann, E., Falk, A., Moliner, A., Lendahl, U., & Ibáñez, C. F. (2003). Cross-talk between the notch and TGF-β signaling pathways mediated by interaction of the notch intracellular domain with Smad3. *The Journal of Cell Biology*, 163(4), 723–728. https://doi.org/10.1083/jcb.200305112.

Boyne, P. J., Lilly, L. C., Marx, R. E., Moy, P. K., Nevins, M., Spagnoli, D. B., & Triplett, R. G. (2005). De novo bone induction by recombinant human bone morphogenetic protein-2 (rhBMP-2) in maxillary sinus floor augmentation. *Journal of Oral and Maxillofacial Surgery*, 63(12), 1693–1707.

Butler, W. T., Ritchie, H., & Bronckers, A. L. J. J. (2003). "Extracellular matrix proteins of dentin." In *Craniofacial Development*, edited by A. L. J. J. Bronckers, vol. 9 of *Frontiers of Oral Biology*, 25–47. Basel: Karger.

Chang, H. H., Chen, I. L., Wang, Y. L., Chang, M. C., Tsai, Y. L., Lan, W. C., Wang, T. M., Yeung, S. Y., & Jeng, J. H. (2020). Regulation of the regenerative activity of dental pulp stem cells from exfoliated deciduous teeth (SHED) of children by TGF-β1 is associated with ALK5/Smad2, TAK1, p38 and MEK/ERK signaling. *Aging*, 12(21), 21253–21272.

Chen, J., Lan, Y., Baek, J. A., Gao, Y., & Jiang, R. (2009). Wnt/beta-catenin signaling plays an essential role in activation of odontogenic mesenchyme during early tooth development. *Developmental Biology*, 334(1), 174–185.

Clevers, H. (2006). Wnt/β-catenin signaling in development and disease. *Cell*, 127(3), 469–480.

Duncan, H. F., Kobayashi, Y., & Shimizu, E. (2018). Growth factors and cell homing in dental tissue regeneration. *Current Oral Health Reports*, 5(4), 276–285. https://doi.org/10.1007/s40496-018-0194-y.

Evans, C. H. (2011). Gene therapy for the regeneration of bone. *Advanced Drug Delivery Reviews*, 64(12), 1331–1340.

Galler, K. M., D'Souza, R. N., Hartgerink, J. D., & Schmalz, G. (2016). Biomimetic approaches in regenerative endodontics: Biomaterials and signaling molecules. *Clinical Oral Investigations*, 20(7), 1489–1503.

Giannobile, W. V., Ryan, S., & Shih, M. S. (1998). Recombinant human osteogenic protein-1 (OP-1) stimulates periodontal wound healing in class III furcation defects. *Journal of Periodontology*, 69(2), 129–137.

James, A. W. (2016). Review of the clinical side effects of bone morphogenetic protein-2. *Tissue Engineering Part B: Reviews*, 22(4), 284–297.

Jung, C., Kim, S., Sun, T., Cho, Y.-B., & Song, M. (2019). Pulp-dentin regeneration: Current approaches and challenges. *Journal of Tissue Engineering*, 10. https://doi.org/10.1177/2041731418819263.

Kim, S. G., Zhou, J., Solomon, C., Zheng, Y., Suzuki, T., Chen, M., Song, S., Jiang, N., Cho, S., & Mao, J. J. (2012). Effects of growth factors on dental stem/progenitor cells. *Journal of Endodontics*, 38(11), 1529–1537.

Li, J., Zhang, C., Huang, X., Xu, F., & Zhang, Y. (2023). TGF-β promotes the proliferation and osteogenic differentiation of dental pulp stem cells: A meta-analysis. *Stem Cells International*, 2023, 1–10.

Liu, F., & Millar, S. E. (2010). Wnt/β-catenin signaling in oral tissue development and disease. *Journal of Dental Research*, 89(4), 318–330.

Liu, X., Chen, X., Sun, L., Zhou, Y., Bai, Y., & Zhang, Q. (2013). BMP2 regulates odontogenic differentiation of dental pulp stem cells through Wnt/β-catenin signaling. *Journal of Cellular Physiology*, 228(12), 2514–2522.

Mao, A. S., & Mooney, D. J. (2015). Regenerative medicine: Current therapies and future directions. *Proceedings of the National Academy of Sciences*, 112(47), 14452–14459.

Miyazono, K., Kamiya, Y., & Morikawa, M. (2010). Bone morphogenetic protein receptors and signal transduction. *Journal of Biochemistry*, 147(1), 35–51.

Moustakas, A., & Heldin, C. H. (2009). The regulation of TGFβ signal transduction. *Development*, 136(22), 3699–3714.

Nakashima, M. (1994). Induction of dentin formation on canine amputated pulp by recombinant human bone morphogenetic proteins (BMP)-2 and -4. *Journal of Dental Research*, 73(9), 1515–1522.

Nakashima, M., & Iohara, K. (2017). Recent progress in regenerative endodontics: Growth factor and stem cell-based therapies. *Journal of Endodontics*, 43(9), S30–S34.

Nakashima, M., & Reddi, A. H. (2003). The application of bone morphogenetic proteins to dental tissue engineering. *Nature Biotechnology*, 21(9), 1025–1032.

Neves, V. C., Babb, R., Chandrasekaran, D., & Sharpe, P. T. (2017). Promotion of natural tooth repair by small molecule GSK3 antagonists. *Scientific Reports*, 7(1), 39654.

Oliveira, É. R., Nie, L., Podstawczyk, D., Allahbakhsh, A., Ratnayake, J., Brasil, D. L., Smith, R. E., Clark, B. S., & Szczepaniak, J. T. (2021). Advances in growth factor delivery for bone tissue engineering. International *Journal of Molecular Sciences*, 22(2), 903.

Park, J. C., Um, S., Kim, Y. I., Kim, S. B., Jung, J. K., & Choi, J. S. (2019). BMP-2 gene delivery-based bone regeneration in dentistry. *International Journal of Molecular Sciences*, 20(10), 2410.

Reddi, A. H., & Huggins, C. B. (1972). Biochemical sequences in the transformation of normal fibroblasts in adolescent rats. *Proceedings of the National Academy of Sciences*, 69(6), 1601–1605.

Schwabe, P., Kluge, K., Wang, H., Bensch, M., Basler, C., Menger, M. D., & Kneser, S. A. (2012). Effect of a novel nonviral gene delivery of BMP-2 on bone healing in a rat fracture model. *Tissue Engineering Part A*, 18(19–20), 2198–2206.

Vainio, S., Karavanova, I., Jowett, A., & Thesleff, I. (1993). Identification of BMP-4 as a signal mediating secondary induction between epithelial and mesenchymal tissues during early tooth development. *Cell*, 75(1), 45–58.

Yamashiro, T., Zheng, L., Shitaku, Y., Saito, M., Tsubakimoto, T., Takada, K., Takano-Yamamoto, T., & Thesleff, I. (2007). Wnt10a regulates dentin sialophosphoprotein mRNA expression and possibly links odontoblast differentiation and tooth morphogenesis. *Differentiation,* 75(5), 452–462. https://doi.org/10.1111/j.1432-0436.2006.00150.x.

Zara, J. N., Siu, R. K., Zhang, X., Shen, J., Ngo, R., Lee, M., Zhang, X., Lee, M., Ting, K., & Soo, C. (2011). High doses of bone morphogenetic protein 2 induce structurally abnormal bone and inflammation in vivo. *Tissue Engineering Part A*, 17(9–10), 1389–1399.

Zhang, R., Cooper, P. R., & Smith, G. (2022). Transforming growth factor-beta1: Effects on odontoblast differentiation and dentin formation. *Frontiers in Physiology*, 13, 1–12.

Zhang, R., Yang, G., Wu, X., Xie, J., Yang, X., Li, T., Lin, Y., & Li, J. (2016). Wnt/β-catenin signaling stimulates the proliferation and odontoblastic differentiation of human dental pulp stem cells. *Cell Biology International*, 40(6), 659–667.

Zhang, Y. E. (2009). Non-Smad pathways in TGF-β signaling. *Cell Research*, 19(1), 128–139. https://doi.org/10.1038/cr.2008.328.

Zhao, H., Feng, J., Ho, T. V., Grimes, W., Urata, M., & Chai, Y. (2020). The role of signaling pathways in tooth development and regeneration. *Development*, 147(23), dev193086.

Index

For Product Safety Concerns and Information please contact our EU representative GPSR@taylorandfrancis.com Taylor & Francis Verlag GmbH, Kaufingerstraße 24, 80331 München, Germany of around 1 GHz, through their spectrum signature. As illustrated in Figures 3.13–3.19, the spectrum of different materials or objects can be identified by the presence or absence of specific frequency components and/or their amplitudes. A combination of several of these diffracting/scattering components forms a unique spectrum signature that can be filtered and applied for recognition.

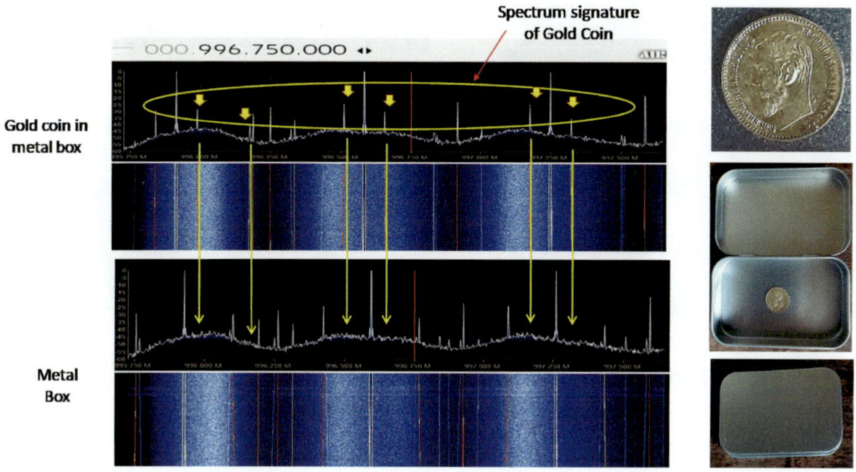

Figure 3.14 Recognition of gold coin inside metal (steel) box by spectrum signature.

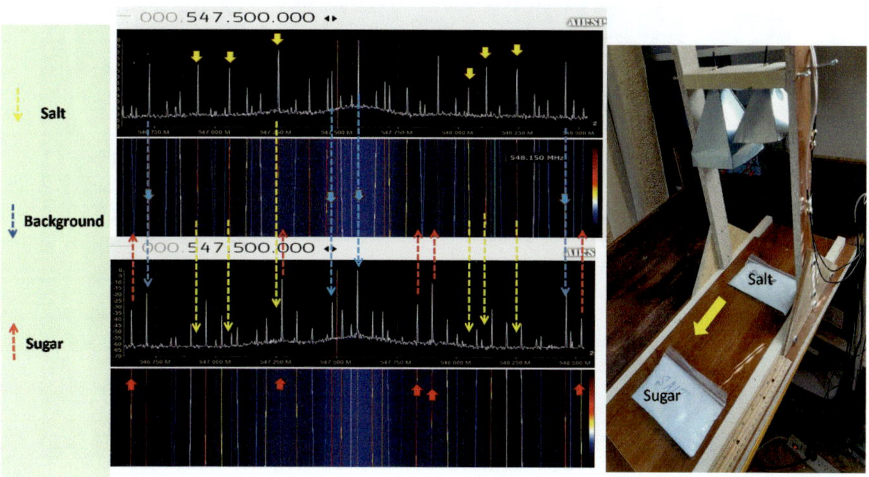

Figure 3.15 Recognition of sugar and salt samples by spectrum signatures.

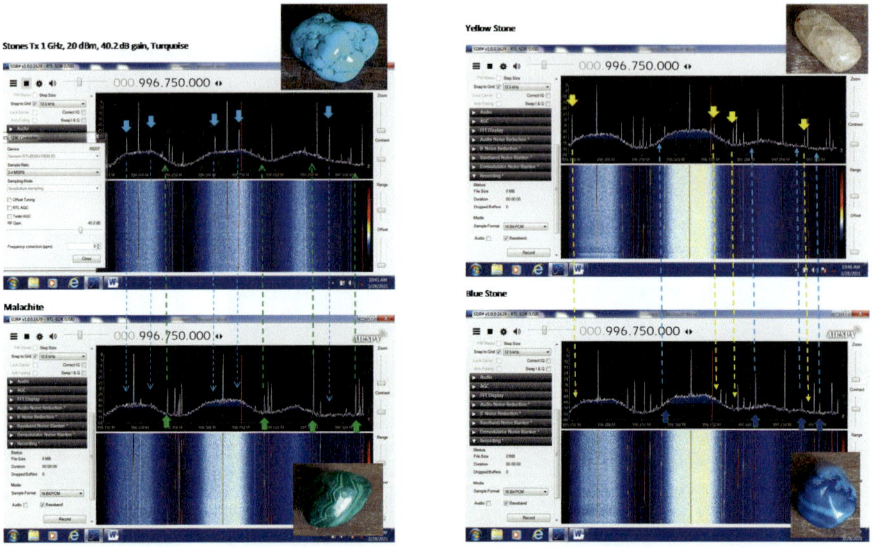

Figure 3.16 Recognition of different stones by spectrum signature.

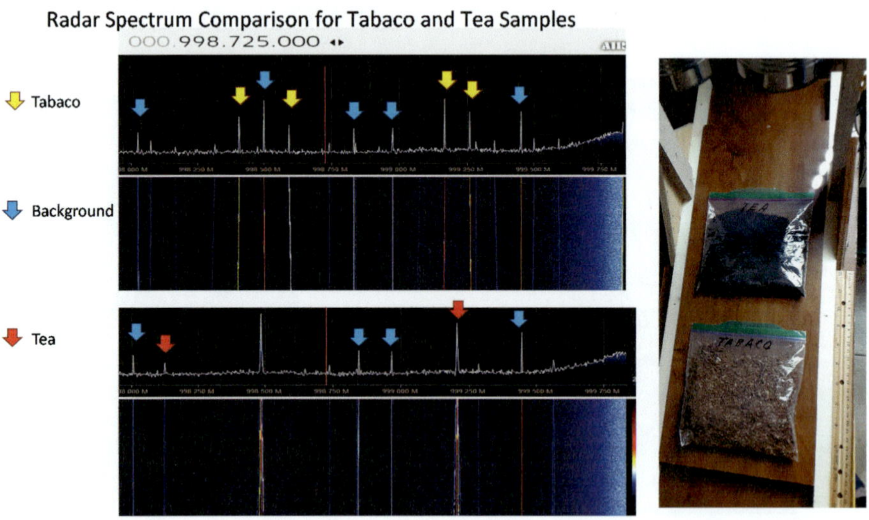

Figure 3.17 Recognition of tobacco and tea by spectrum signature.